Transitions to practice
Essential concepts for health and social care practitioners

For the full range of M&K Publishing books please visit our website:
www.mkupdate.co.uk

Transitions to practice

Essential concepts for health and social care practitioners

•••

Edited by
Teena J. Clouston
Lyn Westcott
Steven W. Whitcombe

Transitions to practice:
Essential concepts for health and social care practitioners
Teena J. Clouston, Lyn Westcott, Steven W. Whitcombe
ISBN: 978-1-910451-08-3
First published 2018

All rights reserved. No part of this publication may be reproduced, stored in a retrieval system, or transmitted in any form or by any means, electronic, mechanical, photocopying, recording or otherwise, without either the prior permission of the publishers or a licence permitting restricted copying in the United Kingdom issued by the Copyright Licensing Agency, 90 Tottenham Court Road, London, W1T 4LP. Permissions may be sought directly from M&K Publishing, phone: 01768 773030, fax: 01768 781099 or email: publishing@mkupdate.co.uk

Any person who does any unauthorised act in relation to this publication may be liable to criminal prosecution and civil claims for damages.

British Library Cataloguing in Publication Data

A catalogue record for this book is available from the British Library

Notice

Clinical practice and medical knowledge constantly evolve. Standard safety precautions must be followed, but, as knowledge is broadened by research, changes in practice, treatment and drug therapy may become necessary or appropriate. Readers must check the most current product information provided by the manufacturer of each drug to be administered and verify the dosages and correct administration, as well as contraindications. It is the responsibility of the practitioner, utilising the experience and knowledge of the patient, to determine dosages and the best treatment for each individual patient. Any brands mentioned in this book are as examples only and are not endorsed by the publisher. Neither the publisher nor the authors assume any liability for any injury and/or damage to persons or property arising from this publication.

To contact M&K Publishing write to:
M&K Update Ltd · The Old Bakery · St. John's Street
Keswick · Cumbria CA12 5AS
Tel: 01768 773030 · Fax: 01768 781099
publishing@mkupdate.co.uk
www.mkupdate.co.uk

Designed and typeset by Mary Blood
Printed in Scotland by Bell & Bain, Glasgow

Contents

List of contributors vii

Preface ix
Heléne Donnelly OBE

Introduction xv
Lyn Westcott, Steven W. Whitcombe and Teena J. Clouston

Section 1
To begin at the beginning: Scaffolding professional practice 1
Introduction by Lyn Westcott

Chapter 1 Professional ethics, registration and fitness to practise 3
Jayne Hancock

Chapter 2 Being professional 17
Janet Kelly and Jacqui Thornton

Chapter 3 Professionalism: A journey from novice to expert practitioner 31
Gary Strong

**Chapter 4: Embracing professionalism:
Becoming a responsible, autonomous practitioner** 45
Lyn Westcott

Section 2
Working together and communication 57
Introduction by Steven W. Whitcombe

Chapter 5 Team working in complex organisations: Principles and practice 59
Tim Lewis

Chapter 6 Partnership working 71
Alison Strode

Chapter 7 Communication in the digital age 85
Fiona Fraser and Katrina Bannigan

Section 3
Quality in practice 97
Introduction by Steven W. Whitcombe

Chapter 8 The political and legal interface with professional practice 99
Heather Hunter

Chapter 9 Duty of quality in times of constraint 113
Sally Abey and Matt Cole

Chapter 10 Research in health and social care practice 127
Steven W. Whitcombe

Section 4
Caring values, spirituality, resilience and the duty of care 137
Introduction by Teena J. Clouston

Chapter 11 Safeguarding vulnerable adults 139
Gareth Morgan

Chapter 12 Safeguarding children 153
Ian Smith

Chapter 13 Evidencing caring values in everyday practice 186
Teena J. Clouston

Chapter 14 The place of spirituality in health and social care practice 189
Melody Cranbourne-Rosser

Chapter 15 The resilient practitioner 205
Stuart Abbott

Epilogue 215
Steven W. Whitcombe, Lyn Westcott and Teena J. Clouston

Index 216

List of contributors

Stuart Abbott MA, BA (Hons), PGCE (FE), FHEA
Learning Development Officer, Learning and Teaching Development Unit, Cardiff Metropolitan University, UK

Sally Abey PhD, PGCert, BSc (Hons), HCPC Registered
Podiatry Programme Lead and Associate Head of School, Marketing and Admissions, School of Health Professions, University of Plymouth; Vice-Dean of Education, College of Podiatry

Katrina Bannigan BD, BSc, PgCLTHE, PhD, SFHEA, MRCOT, HCPC Registered
Associate Professor (Reader) of Occupational Therapy, School of Health Professions, Faculty of Health and Human Sciences, University of Plymouth, UK

Teena J. Clouston PhD, MBA, DipOT, DipCouns, DipArom, CertHyp FHEA, MRCOT, HCPC Registered
Reader, Occupational Therapy and Life Balance/Well-being, School of Healthcare Sciences, College of Biomedical and Life Sciences, Cardiff University, UK

Helené Donnelley OBE, RGN
Ambassador for Cultural Change, Staffordshire and Stoke-on-Trent Partnership NHS Trust

Matthew Cole BSc, DPodM, MChS, HCPC Registered
Podiatry Services Manager, Livewell Southwest CIC, Plymouth, UK

Melody Cranbourne-Rosser MSc, MA, PQDip, PGDip, DipPTh, BSc (Hons), PGCE, FHEA, HCPC Registered
Practitioner Psychologist, Senior Lecturer in Counselling and Therapeutic Practice, School of Psychology and Therapeutic Studies, University of South Wales, UK

Fiona Fraser MSc BSc (Hons), MRCOT, FHEA, HCPC Registered
Practice Placement Lead and Occupational Therapy Lecturer, Faculty of Health and Human Sciences, School of Health Professions, University of Plymouth, UK

Jayne Hancock RGN, ONC, DipN, BSc(Hons) Nursing, PGCE, MSc Education
Lecturer, Nursing, School of Healthcare Sciences, College of Biomedical and Life Sciences, Cardiff University, UK

Heather Hunter MSc, BSc(Hons), FHEA, HCPC Registered
Associate Professor (Senior Lecturer), Academic Lead for Physiotherapy, Faculty of Health and Human Sciences, University of Plymouth, UK

Janet Kelly MSc, DipOT, MRCOT, HCPC Registered
Head of Occupational Therapy Services, Aneurin Bevan University Health Board, Newport, Wales, UK

Tim Lewis MSc, BA (Hons), RODP
Lecturer, Perioperative Professional Head and Placement Coordinator School of Healthcare Sciences, College of Biomedical and Life Sciences, Cardiff University, UK

Gareth Morgan MSc, BA CQSW, PGCE
Lecturer, School of Healthcare Sciences, College of Biomedical and Life Sciences, Cardiff University, UK

Ian D. Smith JP, BSc (Hons), MSc, MCPara
Named Lead Safeguarding, Public Health Wales, Cardiff, UK

Alison Strode DSocSci, MSc, BSc(Open), DPodM, CertHE, MChS
Chief Therapies Advisor (Acting), Directorate of Health Policy, Health and Social Service Group, Welsh Government

Gary Strong MClined, PGDipClined, PGCE, BA (Hons), MCP, MPA, HCPC Registered
Paramedic, writer and researcher; Former Programme Lead BSc(Hons) Paramedicine, University of Plymouth, UK

Jacqui Thornton MSc, DipOT, PGCE, HCPC Registered
Practice Development and Education Lead for Occupational Therapy, Anuerin Bevan University Health Board, Newport, UK

Lyn Westcott MSc, BSc, DipCOT, FHEA, MRCOT, HCPC Registered
Associate Professor (Senior Lecturer), Associate Head of School of Health Professions: Internationalisation, Academic Lead Occupational Therapy, Faculty of Health and Human Sciences, University of Plymouth, UK

Steven W. Whitcombe Ed.D, MSc, BScOT(Hons), BA(Hons), PGCE(PCET), FHEA, MRCOT, HCPC Registered
Senior Lecturer, Occupational Therapy and Health Professional Education, School of Healthcare Sciences, College of Biomedical and Life Sciences, Cardiff University, UK

The editorial team would like to gratefully acknowledge the invaluable contribution of Patricia McClure, EdD, Med, PGDipEd, PGCUT, BSc(Hons), DipCOT, MRCOT, SFHEA, FCHERP, Associate Head of School Health Sciences, Ulster University, HCPC Registered, in offering her time and expertise to review key chapters in the book. Thank you.

Preface

Helené Donnelly OBE

I am pleased to write the preface for this important book as I feel that the quality of practice and care in the NHS and social care systems needs to be challenged and improvements made where needed. Human dignity, respect and care for both patients and staff are fundamental to everything we do in the NHS and social care. I believe this book can help all health and social care workers make the transition into this type of healthy working culture.

After the tragic cases of poor care at the Mid Staffordshire Foundation Trust Hospital came to public attention in 2010, it was clear that the NHS needed a drastic culture shift. The suffering of patients at the hospital resulted from a widespread negative culture and a failure on the part of senior staff to listen to the legitimate complaints of staff and patients over a long period of time. I strongly believe that much-needed change hinges on shaping working environments where health care professionals are encouraged to demonstrate openness and transparency.

The Francis Report (2013) revealed that much of what occurred at the Mid Staffordshire Foundation Trust (Mid Staffs) was due to historic and entrenched mismanagement and the unprofessional conduct of some staff. In fact, the legacy of the failings at Mid Staffs should lead to widespread cultural change throughout the NHS, health and social care systems. I have always strongly believed that what occurred at Mid Staffs, was not a unique, isolated incident. Many of the problems at Mid Staffs will have occurred in other wards, units, clinics and hospitals throughout the country at the same time. Sadly, many such incidents predated the Francis Report (2013), and similar tragedies continue to come to light.

Since the Francis inquiry (and the publication of several reports on the events at Mid Staffs), positive steps have been taken towards creating a culture of openness in the NHS. These measures have included the introduction of a statutory Duty of Candour and the appointment of Freedom to Speak Up Guardians, changes to the way unions respond to concerns raised by their members and changes to professional regulations.

Openness on the part of staff is crucial in order to protect patient safety and prevent needless harm; and these values must be embedded across the entire health and care system. Most professionals working in the health and social care services already know that they need to be honest about mistakes they make, and constantly strive to do the best job possible. Health and social care is often delivered in intense environments by hard-pressed staff. By truly listening to the staff who deliver this care when they have concerns, most harm can and should be prevented. When executing their Duty of Candour, staff must be supported and encouraged by the organisations they work for. In order to embed such a culture change, it is imperative that action is taken to address issues as soon as legitimate concerns have been raised, and feedback must be given to all those involved. This will promote the positive impact of raising concerns and, crucially, will improve patient and staff safety.

I can write about this from personal experience, as I became increasingly worried about the welfare of patients and staff whilst working at Mid Staffs hospital. Due to this and the poor experience I had, I am well aware of how difficult and daunting it is to raise such concerns.

As a newly qualified nurse in 2002, I commenced a staff nurse development rotation at Mid Staffordshire hospital. Having trained elsewhere, I went to Mid Staffs with fresh eyes and looked forward to nursing in a hospital close to my home. I had chosen a critical care programme, which rotated every six months between acute units and wards over a two-year period to enhance specialist skills and knowledge. I spent the first year working on an acute respiratory ward and then on the Acute Cardiac Unit. This was a particularly good unit to work on and gave me an opportunity to develop my nursing skills and knowledge whilst delivering excellent care to patients. The staff were knowledgeable, professional, kind and caring.

I later moved to the Medical Assessment Unit. This was an extremely busy unit with a very high turnover of patients during each shift. The unit was not as well staffed as it should have been, but the staff worked well together, often under pressure, and delivered the best possible care and treatment for patients.

At this point, I successfully applied for a permanent post in the neighbouring Accident and Emergency (A&E) department, and in 2004 I started work as a staff nurse. Almost immediately I began to have concerns about the staffing of the department. It was clear that there were not enough nurses or doctors working in A&E for us to deliver safe and effective care. The situation was made worse by a high turnover of staff and high levels of staff sickness. For instance, there was often no triage nurse available to assess patient need and priority upon arrival, which put patient safety at risk.

The use of agency staff was not permitted, as it was deemed too expensive; for similar reasons, bank staff were also seldom used. If bank staff were permitted, they would usually be from the pool of existing A&E staff. This meant that already exhausted staff were returning to complete extra shifts. On the rare occasions when external bank staff were permitted to work in A&E this still did not relieve much of the pressure because they were not familiar with the way the department worked, and needed staff to show them what to do. Unfortunately, their presence neither alleviated the pressure the existing staff were under nor improved the patients' experiences.

In addition to low staffing levels, staff were not receiving adequate mandatory and statutory training. There was little or no professional development or supervision; and the department lacked vital equipment needed to deliver specific drugs and other treatments. Facilities required to ensure patients' dignity and privacy were lacking. There were not enough blankets to keep patients warm, nor enough commodes to assist patients to go to the toilet.

Furthermore, there were too few beds/trolleys in the department to examine patients on and make them comfortable. The flow of patients through the hospital was often disrupted and delayed. This meant patients in A&E could not be transferred to an appropriate ward within the four-hour time limit.

It soon became clear that the pressure of the four-hour wait in A&E (i.e. the need to discharge each patient exactly four hours after admission to the department) took priority over their care and treatment. Pressure from management meant that patients were prioritised in time order (so as not to breach the four-hour time limit), rather than according to their physical or emotional needs. Some staff felt bullied and intimidated by the management. This, in turn, led to some staff members falsifying patient records to make it look as if patients had left the department within four hours, when in reality they had remained in A&E for up to an hour or more in some cases.

The creation of a Clinical Decisions Unit (CDU) was an attempt to manage the flow of patients more effectively and prevent patients remaining in A&E longer than four hours. The CDU was intended to be a specifically designated area for patients to await a clinical decision as to whether they were to be discharged home or admitted. Strict criteria stated that patients who were admitted to this unit must have been seen and assessed by an A&E doctor, they must not require cardiac monitoring and they must not be vulnerable or require observation.

However, these and other directions were not adhered to. The CDU was simply an old, disused A&E operating theatre which was quickly fitted out with four beds. There was no natural light and no appropriate disabled toilet or washing facilities. The unit was situated at the bottom of a long corridor within the A&E department and was very isolated. No extra staff were provided to staff the unit and it was an added responsibility for the existing A&E staff.

Patients could not understand why they were remaining in the A&E department well over the four hours and sometimes for days. Vulnerable, confused older patients were left on their own, without adequate safety precautions. This resulted in some falling out of bed, causing injury and distress.

Patients were often left lying in their own urine or faeces and staff were either too busy to attend to them, or by their own admission, 'could not be bothered'. The lack of dignity, care and compassion shown by some staff was astounding.

The pressure to discharge patients who had not been adequately medically assessed (either because the patient was going to breach the four-hour time limit or because there wasn't enough space in the department) became dangerous. Often patients were treated as an inconvenience and a nuisance. Many who had been discharged without proper assessment, examinations and treatment had to return to A&E; some tragically died.

The unprofessional behaviour of some staff created a culture of fear and intimidation. Many staff worked exceptionally hard and cared a great deal. However, some staff in senior positions dismissed concerns that were raised. They would bully subordinates, using menacing, ridiculing, threatening and intimidating behaviour. They would apply pressure to doctors to discharge patients before it was safe to do so, and would threaten staff who did not falsify patient documents pertaining to the four-hour wait. Consequently, patients were harmed, staff were negatively affected and much-needed improvements to the department were never realised.

I persisted in raising concerns internally, which were initially ignored. Eventually an internal investigation was undertaken. This was both corrupt and ineffective and subsequently nothing changed. I therefore began to make my concerns known outside the organisation. I attempted to raise my concerns with the Health Care Commission (now the Care Quality Commission (CQC)) and with my Union, the Royal College of Nursing (RCN). Unfortunately, these efforts came to nothing and I began to feel very discouraged.

In 2008, I left the Mid Staffordshire Foundation Trust to work as a Nurse Practitioner in a neighbouring Trust. Although I had left the organisation, I remained very concerned about the patients and staff who were potentially still suffering. Consequently, I began to raise my concerns with local MPs and campaign groups. This resulted in my giving evidence at the first Francis Independent Inquiry and then at the Francis Public Inquiry. I was later called to give further evidence at a Nursing and Midwifery Council (NMC) Fitness to Practise hearing, which led to two senior nurses being struck off the NMC register.

When I spoke out about the appalling standards of care and low staff morale at Stafford Hospital, I was at first ignored and then threatened. I therefore know how isolating, frustrating and frightening it can be to speak up. Many factors can prevent staff from speaking up. Some fear that their career prospects will suffer; some fear losing their job; some fear being discredited; some are reluctant because it may require them to speak up against friends and colleagues and some are concerned about the potential negative impact on their relationships with friends and family in the local community.

These are all understandable fears and real potential barriers for some. However, raising concerns needs to be normalised so that it is no longer stressful and emotionally draining. Ultimately staff must have faith in the knowledge that they are raising legitimate concerns because it is their professional duty to do so, and that they will be treated fairly. Staff need to feel empowered and enabled to raise concerns before these issues affect patient care.

As a senior nurse with over 19 years of experience working in health and social care, I very much welcome the initiatives put in place since the Francis Report (2013). I am especially proud of the development of Freedom to Speak Up Guardians. I believe that, if these roles are embedded correctly, and fully supported, they will make a real difference to how staff raise concerns. However, there is always more to be done and we must never become complacent. The information and soft intelligence gained from having a Guardian in place will help prevent problems reoccurring in the future. This should help to encourage and support staff to make positive improvements to the services and care they deliver.

If we do not respect and look after our staff, how can we expect them to look after patients and service users? Low staff morale leads to increased stress, errors and sickness absence. This will clearly have a negative impact on the delivery of good-quality, safe care of patients.

In an ever-changing NHS and social care system, we must ensure that staff are consulted and their opinions respected when implementing change. Many staff report feeling devalued and disrespected as change happens *to* them, rather than *with* them. These staff members can often see that proposed changes will not be sustainable or conducive to ensuring patient or staff safety. Having had personal experience of trying to raise concerns whilst at the Mid Staffordshire Foundation Trust and having been bullied and threatened as a result, I feel compelled to use my experience to highlight these issues and help improve the process of raising such concerns at a national level.

As qualified health or social care professionals and students, you will be aware that you too have a duty to speak up and raise concerns should you have them. In order to do this, you firstly need to be clear and confident about identifying what constitutes professional concern, and secondly be clear and confident about knowing how to actually raise your concern. Being a confident and competent professional means being prepared to act in this way, and know that it is the right thing to do.

In conclusion, we should all be very proud of the NHS and our social care provision and should be working in health and social care precisely because we do care! Unfortunately, though, there may be times when we see poor standards of care, or misconduct or unacceptable behaviour and we all have a duty to speak out about it. Nothing is ever perfect, but I would like to see an NHS that truly encourages and supports its staff in raising concerns, rather than at best paying lip service, or at worst intimidating and ignoring them.

We can create and maintain a culture that *expects* people to raise concerns when things are not right, and views it as abnormal for them not to do so. As the NHS and social care system is in a constant state of change, practitioners in these fields have to be prepared to deal with a wide range of professional issues. This requires knowledge, resilience, compassion and genuine empathy in order to uphold the values that should be central for all workers in these areas. This is what you must maintain, irrespective of any transitions you move through in your career, whether you progress from student to qualified practitioner, novice to senior practitioner, or practitioner to manager. I hope this book will help you, wherever you are on this journey, as you are the future of service provision and the future must be one of care and respect.

Introduction

Lyn Westcott, Steven W. Whitcombe and Teena J. Clouston

This book emerged from our awareness of the increasing complexity of health and social care systems in the UK and the skills that professionals have to acquire to meet their demands. As editors of this book working in British universities, we particularly wanted to support the transitions of students and early career practitioners in their practice and help them find their way as professionals in health and social care in the four UK nations. These systems have been in a constant state of change throughout our own careers and this is set to continue, so we knew that the text would need to help you, the readers, understand important concepts that would support your development as professionals in a 'moving landscape'. The book is therefore not a guide to the changing context of health and social care, although inevitably a snapshot of those changes will appear within it. Instead, this book has been compiled to offer personal and professional strategies that will help you develop and flourish in this changing field of work.

Fundamental to achieving this is the ability to pass through key transitional phases confidently and successfully. When we talk about transitions, we mean moving between distinct steps that mark your progression as a health and social care professional. These could be personal steps, linked to your career progression; they may concern the evolution of your profession; or they may be organisational changes, like the major UK-wide agenda of aligning the work of health and social care which is currently steering service developments.

Some of these transitions will be linked to personal aspirations, technological developments, changes to funding systems, new evidence that guides practice or other (sometimes political) drivers to enhance quality and standards of practice. Consider, for example, the critical impact of the Francis Report (2013) which highlighted serious shortcomings in practice, quality of care, personal integrity of NHS staff and how policy could over-ride the importance of human compassion when working with vulnerable people. You may want to read the preface for a first-hand account of the personal impact of the events of Mid Staffordshire and how one professional responded to this. This report, and people's responses to it, have enforced significant change and highlighted the importance of successful transitions amongst individual practitioners. In addition, organisations that offer health and social care services have had to adapt, driven by a revised political and public mandate that values dignity, care and compassion above unrealistic targets and financial constraints.

In this book, we focus on important areas that influence our practice and affect transitions at a personal, organisational, professional and political level. The contributors are all specialists representing a wide range of professions across the health and social care sectors in the UK. Some are practitioners; others are managers, policy makers, researchers and educators. All are experts in their own field and share a passion to improve services and ease the transitions involved.

To assist the reader, the book has been divided into four main sections, each with an introduction to help you plan your learning.

The first section 'To begin at the beginning: Scaffolding professional practice' contains four chapters exploring fundamental aspects of professionalism. These include the implications of registration, expectations of a professional in their practice, and how to sustain professionalism over a long period of time.

The second section 'Working together and communication' addresses the importance of communication for effective health and social care practice. This is an area that is subject to continual evolution and change. Through examination of team and partnership working, specific aspects of working life for the health or social care professional in complex organisations are considered. This section finishes with a chapter on communication in the digital age and raises some personal issues to think about as a professional in an instant communication-rich society.

The third section 'Quality in practice' has three chapters focusing on drivers that steer the changes in health and social care services and how these are implemented. With chapters on political systems and mechanisms in the four UK nations, achieving quality with limited resources and the role of research in health and social care, the authors of this section help readers to consider how their practice is influenced at a national level to achieve high standards within budgetary constraints.

The final section 'Understanding values and the duty of care' returns to a more personal agenda for practitioners concerning our interaction with the people we work with. Chapters on safeguarding adults and children provide some thought-provoking content on our duties to some of the most vulnerable people in society. Other authors raise issues about caring values, revisiting how essential these are, and what happens if things go wrong. A chapter on spirituality in health and social care practice explores a dimension of your practice that you may not have considered but is always there within health and social care work. Finally, there is a chapter that looks at protecting yourself as a practitioner in an emotionally demanding area of work. These self-preservation strategies are essential to ensure that you remain healthy, strong and resilient throughout your career.

The book finishes with an Epilogue, in which we as editors draw together its key messages. We link these to the concept of transitions and highlight the importance of the interconnectedness of the themes described throughout the book in terms of health and social care practice. This final contribution suggests how you might wish to take these messages forward in your own career journey.

As you would expect, many of the chapters in this book share common themes and, where appropriate, there are cross-references to other parts of the book. Each contributor has outlined a number of specific learning outcomes for their chapter. It is recommended that you read these outcomes carefully before each full chapter in order to maximise your own learning. The chapters also contain reflective questions to help you apply the discussion to your own experiences and practice. They have been designed to challenge you and help you embed the content into your own professional journey and the important transitions you may undergo within it.

Whilst some of these reflective questions may seem very general, the depth of inquiry they prompt will develop over time – because you will undergo transitions in your career and, in addition, the systems you work in (like the NHS or social care services), will be in a constant state of change. Bearing this in mind, it may be helpful to keep a note of your responses to the questions and revisit them later in your study or career to see how things have developed and altered in your own thinking. It will be interesting to track your appreciation of the meaning of the concepts involved and how they impact on your practice. Reflections of this type have the added value of helping you monitor your own professional development and giving you feedback on your own personal transitions in the career journey.

Please note: The contributions in this book reflect the personal opinions of each of the authors. They do not represent the views of the organisations that employ them. The terms 'patient', 'client' and 'service user' are used interchangeably in the book and represent the personal choice of the author. In all cases, these terms are used to describe the people accessing health and social care services.

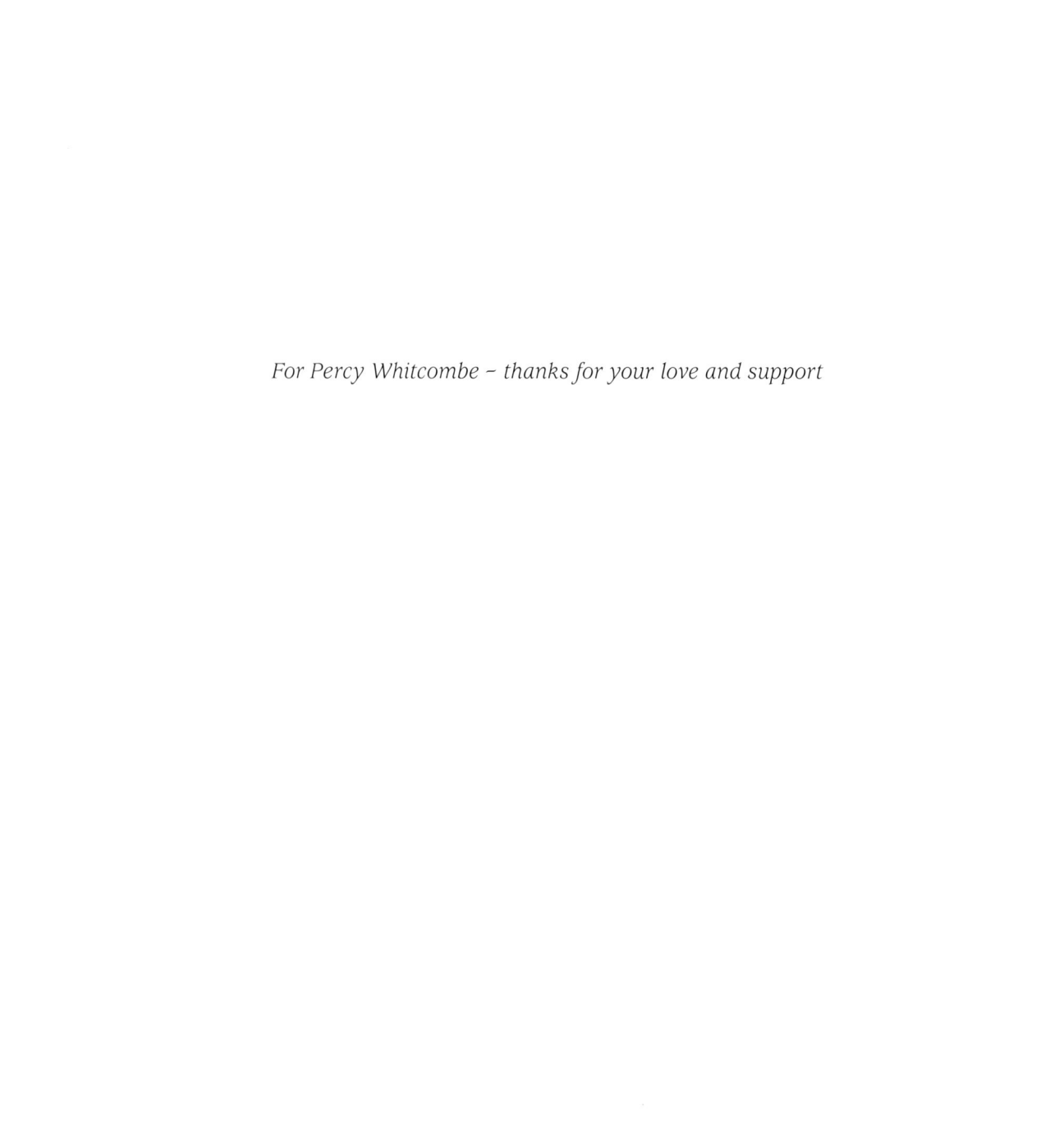

For Percy Whitcombe – thanks for your love and support

Section 1
To begin at the beginning: Scaffolding professional practice

Introduction
by Lyn Westcott

This initial section of the book examines some fundamental concepts that underpin the more personal elements of professionalism for effective, high-quality health and social care practice.

All professionals working in health and social care systems in the UK have accepted the need for their practice to be subject to wider quality systems and frameworks. These frameworks ensure that every practitioner operates within baselines of safety and competence in order to protect the public and the scope of their practice. This has not developed by chance, but out of a need for effective regulation and scrutiny following a series of shocking failures by professionals, such as that at the Mid Staffordshire Hospital described in the Preface. Alongside this, each new professional develops their skills and thinking to meet society's expectations of their professional role, as well as their own expectations of themselves as a professional practitioner.

This section takes a dual approach to these fundamental issues concerning the concept of professionalism. One approach is to look at the systems that monitor professional practice; the other considers the more personal journey that guides, develops and sustains people when they become newly qualified professionals. This section therefore explores aspects of the key transition from layperson to professional practitioner. Some of the chapters describe systems and expectations that all practitioners need to understand and abide by. Others consider how individuals can embrace the challenges of becoming a professional practitioner. They look at each person entering the professional world and gaining an understanding of their role and obligations within that world. This section thus provides an underlying structure or scaffolding for the later sections of the book. It is a useful section for students, new practitioners or those mentoring or educating students within practice settings.

Chapter 1 sets the scene by outlining the importance of professional ethics, registration systems and fitness to practice procedures in health and social care. Drawing on the lessons of critical incidents from the recent past, the author outlines how systems such as registration and maintenance of ethical standards by professionals ensure the safety of the general public, including the importance of raising concerns about services when working within them. The chapter finishes by posing some reflective questions on how all this works on the ground and challenges the reader to reflect on their role in maintaining ethical standards.

Chapter 2 is authored by two NHS service managers and discusses professionalism in terms of expectations concerning specific professional behaviours within practice settings, especially for students. The chapter challenges the reader by raising specific examples where professionalism might be questioned through behaviours seen in the workplace. It also highlights situations where expectations might differ between academic settings and placement settings. The chapter concludes by asking readers to reflect on a framework of issues that contribute towards professional behaviours.

Chapter 3 takes a very personal approach to considering the journey towards professionalism, making the transition from novice student to more expert practitioner. Using an engaging script-based writing style, the author examines how students move through the challenges of becoming a professional in how they think and behave both within and outside their work. The personal journeys of four health profession students are linked to theory and guidance relevant to novice practitioners becoming more expert professionals. Using reflective questions, the chapter finally challenges the reader to consider their own level of professionalism and how this will change as their career progresses.

Finally, **Chapter 4** considers the issues that contribute to people becoming and remaining responsible and autonomous professionals. This chapter encourages the reader to consider their own resources and how these can help them maintain professional growth against a background of persistent change in health and social care, as well as offering some tips on how to do this. The challenge of fitting in development activities is raised and the reader is encouraged to think about remaining resilient to avoid 'burnout'. The chapter ends by asking the reader to evaluate how they might ensure their own development is maintained and learn from robust role models around them.

In order to get the most from these chapters we ask that you really engage with and reflect on the questions and practical exercises you will find in them. It is only through an honest and meaningful exploration of your own beliefs and values that you will gain the full benefit of this book

Chapter 1
Professional ethics, registration and fitness to practise

Jayne Hancock

Learning outcomes
By the end of this chapter you will be able to understand:
- The importance of professional ethics within health and social care
- The role of professional bodies in health and social care and how regulatory processes assist in maintaining key standards for performance and ethics
- Fitness to practise and the importance of health and social care regulation in ensuring the safety of the general public
- How to apply ethical principles to practice and recognise personal responsibility in raising and escalating concerns, also known as 'whistleblowing'.

Introduction

Professional ethics can be defined as 'matters of right and wrong conduct, good and bad qualities of character and the professional responsibilities attached to relationships in a work context' (Banks 2012, p. 7).

Practitioners in health and social care settings work in partnership with multidisciplinary teams, individuals (as clients/patients) and families, usually at times when they are at their most vulnerable. The common aim across the whole health and social care sector is to provide high-quality care and support to ensure the best interests of the individual are central to the provision of an excellent service. It is therefore essential that health and social care practitioners understand the importance of professional ethics across the health and social care spectrum, and how professional ethics form the cornerstone of professional regulation, registration and fitness to practise.

Professional ethics

Ethics is essentially the study of morals and the nature of morality. Morals are the values, principles, rules and practices by which people live, based on socially accepted principles of right and wrong (Melia 2014). A moral individual may be described as honest, righteous, respectable, decent, virtuous, upstanding, high-minded and law-abiding. However, rules of behaviour mean different things to different people depending upon their own life experiences. Ellis (2015) recognised the importance of personal and professional ethics being compatible with each other – because the way we behave in our everyday lives, as individuals, is inextricably linked to our professional behaviour.

> ### Case study 1.1
> An individual who is drunk and disorderly at a football match is arrested after assaulting a member of the public and stealing from them. During court proceedings, they are identified as being a health care professional in a responsible role, caring for vulnerable adults.
> - In this situation, how might their behaviour impact on their role as a health or social care professional?
> - Highlight the concerns this person's employer and the public may have.
> - Reflect on how you would feel, having to work with this person.

Professional ethics are the accepted standard of personal and professional behaviour expected of a member of a profession. Ethics are fundamental to the professional practice of health and social care practitioners who need to behave in an ethically acceptable way. The World Health Organisation (2011) identify ethics as 'moral principles, values and standards of conduct', recognising the way they are inextricably linked to health care delivery, professional integrity and data handling – especially while working with members of the public when they are at their most vulnerable.

There are a number of ethical principles that health and social care professionals need to consider in their practice:

- *Autonomy* or self-rule is the capacity to think, decide and act freely and independently
- *Beneficence* is the promotion of what is best for the client or service user
- *Non-maleficence* is the avoidance of harm to the client or service user

- *Justice* is fairness within health care; 'to each according to his need' without discrimination, a balance of time and resources.

These points are supported by *veracity* (accuracy), *privacy, truthfulness, confidentiality* and *fidelity* (duty of care) (Seedhouse 2009; Beauchamp & Childress 2013).

At the centre of health care ethics is the individual's own sense of right and wrong and our beliefs about it. These influence how we act, and define the moral choices we make. Moral choices can be influenced by values and beliefs about life, health, suffering and death. Individual ethical practice may drive behaviour and decisions made, but professional ethics are an indispensable and inherent element of health care today because they provide key standards of conduct, performance and ethics for health care practitioners (Beauchamp & Childress 2013, Melia 2015). This point was made as long ago as 1863 by Florence Nightingale, when she stated: 'It may seem a strange principle to enunciate as the very first requirement in a hospital that it should do the sick no harm' (p. 9).

Sound ethical principles have been established for health and social care practitioners by their professional bodies, which have developed codes of conduct and standards of conduct, performance and ethics. These reinforce professionalism, provide guidance for individual practitioners and employers and, most importantly, define the standards that patients/clients and members of the general public can expect from *all* health and social care professionals.

The core values inherent in an ethical code are non-negotiable. They provide a non-discretionary set of guiding principles for health and social care professionals, based on the need for *honesty, integrity* and *personal responsibility*. These documents provide a set of expectations and principles for measuring conduct and personal responsibility, developed by the professions to protect the public through regulation. A health care professional can be judged by these standards in relation to fitness for practice – for instance, *The Code of Ethics for Social Work* (The Policy, Ethics and Human Rights Committee 2012) and *The Code* (Nursing and Midwifery Council 2015). Codes of conduct are seen as a sign of good practice and have been developed voluntarily within some sectors as guidance for employers, workers and the public. A prime example for non-qualified staff is *The Code of Conduct for Health Care Support Workers and Adult Social Care Workers in England*, developed by Skills for Care (2013).

Since the millennium, there have been an increasing number of concerning disclosures relating to health and social care standards. These have included shocking revelations in the press, highlighting patterns of serious abuse, neglect, poor standards of care, high mortality rates and multiple care failings in a number of health and social care arenas. Some of these revelations have led to independent reviews (see Chapter 13 for more on this). The resulting extensive inquiries (such as the Winterbourne Review

2012, the Francis Report 2013, the Morecambe Bay Investigation 2015, and the Andrews Report 2014) identified appalling negligence at all levels. Examples included poor hygiene standards, food and drink left out of reach, poor documentation, inappropriate pain management and a number of other issues. Consequently, many patients/clients and their families, may, through personal experience of poor health or social care provision, have lost confidence in the professionals in these areas. Moreover, the general public are rightly concerned that these shocking patterns of negligence are more widespread than we known, and that these reported failings may just be the tip of the iceberg.

Hughes (2008) recognised that in today's complex care system, many different factors can influence professional standards of care. These include the work environment, complex patient needs and care processes, unsupportive organisational culture, limited resources, and a lack of standardised procedures. All these factors can adversely affect health and social care standards; and the way professional practitioners recognise and address such issues is inextricably linked to the ethical codes that guide practice.

As consumers of health and social care, members of the public need to be assured that every health and social care practitioner recognises that they are professionally accountable for their own actions and works to maintain high standards where openness, transparency and candour are cornerstones of everyday practice. Ethical standards must ensure that the public are protected and that, through statutory regulation of professional bodies, the government can ensure appropriate regulation of health care providers.

The regulatory process within health care in the UK

In order to protect the public and enhance public confidence, the UK government, through statute (law), regulates a vast majority of the health/social care workforce. Legislation such as the Health Act (1999), the Nursing and Midwifery Order (2001) and the Health and Care Professions Order (2015) sets an operational framework that can only be changed through legislation. Each regulatory body is accountable to the Privy Council, the Department of Health and the devolved administrations and the Professional Standards Authority (PSA).

The PSA is a proactive, independent body that is accountable to the UK Parliament. It oversees the UK health and social care regulatory bodies in order to protect the public and act as a strong, independent voice. It works to share good practice, knowledge and research to ensure safety, improve quality of care and promote the health, and well-being of the public. The role of the PSA includes raising the standards of regulation through:

- Carrying out annual performance reviews of the nine professional bodies
- Setting standards for organisations holding voluntary registers for health and social care and accrediting those that meet the standards

- Reviewing fitness to practise committee final decisions made by the professional bodies; these can then be appealed and referred on to court if the sanctions are considered unduly lenient or if it is in the public interest to do so
- Auditing fitness to practise processes within each professional body
- Presenting the annual report and accounts to the UK Parliament, Scottish Parliament, Welsh Government and Northern Ireland Assembly.

Professional standards and regulation are about making sure that individual practitioners within health and social care meet the key regulatory standards of their profession. To achieve and maintain registration, health and social care professionals must meet specific standards of education, competence and conduct. Registration with a professional body is an important measurement of an individual's competence and suitability for their role, and their fitness to practise, which both the public and employers recognise.

There are twelve health and social care regulators that abide by legal frameworks to oversee the health and social care professions. These regulators are required to do four things:

1. Set the professional standards of conduct, performance and ethics that health and social care professionals must meet in order to register and practise

2. Set standards for professional proficiency in relation to the quality of education and training to ensure students have the skills to practise safely and to set standards for behaviour and health

3. Keep and maintain a public register of professionals who have demonstrated that they have met key professional regulation standards to enter and remain on the register

4. Investigate complaints regarding conduct or competence about people on the register and decide, through fitness to practise procedures, whether the individual should be allowed to continue to practise.

Setting the standards for conduct

Standards of conduct, performance and ethics provide a framework of set expectations for the behaviour and conduct of a registrant. They are important because they outline what the public can expect of the practitioner in relation to their behaviour when providing care or treatment. For example, the Health and Care Professions Council (2016) states that registrants must:

- Promote and protect the interests of service users and carers
- Communicate appropriately and fairly
- Work within the limits of their knowledge and skills
- Delegate appropriately

- Respect confidentiality
- Manage risk
- Report concerns about safety
- Be open when things go wrong
- Be honest and trustworthy
- Keep records of their work.

These standards regulating health and social care professions are consistent with standards developed by other regulatory bodies. The provision of a standard gives the regulatory body a mechanism by which health and social care practitioners can be measured. When the character of a professional is questioned (through registration or fitness to practise), these organisations need to see if the registrant has met, or fallen short, of the standard. The professional standards ensure parity and equity of treatment for every individual practitioner and assure the public that appropriate action is being taken.

Professional proficiency

Each regulator sets the standards of proficiency for a profession. For example, the Nursing and Midwifery Council (2010) sets the standards for pre-registration nursing education in the UK. The regulator aims to establish a 'threshold standard' that students must meet to complete their education/training and register with their professional body. The standards for the quality of the education programme determine the programme content, learning outcomes and assessment criteria and are underpinned by specific requirements, such as the length of the course, the theory and clinical hours required whilst on the course, the scope of practice, the required knowledge, and the skills and experience to practise lawfully, safely and effectively. Each regulator has audit mechanisms in place to ensure that the required standards are being met by the educational institutions and their practice partners.

Maintenance of the register

A number of health and social care professionals are regulated by statute (law) and must register with the regulating body in order to practise. Other parts of the health and social care workforce participate in voluntary registration programmes. Each regulator is responsible for the integrity of the live register to enhance public trust, recognise the professional qualifications and unite the profession. In this way, registration not only protects the public but also indicates competence and suitability to practise. Notably, it is the responsibility of each practitioner to ensure they do not practise without registration. However, practitioners put themselves at significant legal risk if they do not comply, as it is illegal to practise without registration and is a criminal offence to falsely represent yourself as a member of a profession. Employers are required to ensure that their employees are qualified and competent to perform the duties required of the post held. Checking their registration status can help ensure that this is the case.

Investigate complaints

Each regulator must have in place a system whereby the public or employer can raise concerns if a practitioner's skills, knowledge, good health or good character fall below the expected standards of the professional body. Allegations or concerns raised are investigated in relation to the following areas: misconduct, lack of competence, lack of English language, criminal behaviour and serious ill-health. Each regulator has a process in place to investigate allegations and take appropriate action to protect the public. The PSA scrutinises this process to ensure it is fair, equitable and maintains public safety as a core value.

Fitness to practise

In this section, fitness to practise (FTP) will be described and the role of the professional body, health or social care provider and individual practitioner will be explored; short case studies with reflective points will be utilised to support learning. The importance of *openness* and *honesty* with reference to key legislation, such as *duty of candour*, will be discussed to enable readers to reflect on their professional behaviour and recognise their personal responsibility in terms of raising and escalating concerns and whistleblowing.

What is fitness to practise?

Someone who is fit to practise has the skills, knowledge and character to work safely and effectively with patients or clients. A simple way to remember this is as follows:

Skills + Knowledge + Character = Safe, Effective, Practice

Health and social care regulators have a duty to protect the public and the public has a right to expect that their health or social care professional is fit to practise. If a registered professional does not meet the standards expected of them (i.e. those that are clearly outlined within the professional regulator's code of conduct), they can be removed from the register or their practice can be restricted.

Information on an individual practitioner, be it a complaint or allegation, may come from a number of sources:

- The employer
- The public
- A fellow professional
- Self-referral
- Investigating authority, e.g. the police

- A report from another regulator
- A patient or client
- The monitoring arm of the regulator itself.

Health and social care students on a programme of study that leads directly to, or that satisfies a necessary condition of, a professional qualification are also required to meet the standards of the professional body. The professional body may have guidance on professional conduct, good health and character specifically for students; that must be adhered to and may need to be evidenced during audit procedures. All approved educational institutions are accountable to the regulatory body.

The professional body/regulator requires every Approved Educational Institution (AEI) to have a robust system of fitness to practise procedures in place. As such students may face AEI disciplinary mechanisms where their behaviour does not meet the required standards. The AEI disciplinary procedures may result in removal from the programme or other sanctions and potentially lead to being rendered as not fit to be admitted to that profession.

Information on an individual student, be it a complaint or allegation may come from a number of parties:

- The AEI
- The public
- A fellow student
- Self-referral
- Investigating authority such as the police
- A patient or client
- A clinical educator.

Duty of candour

Regulation 20: Duty of candour (Care Quality Commission 2015) states that all health and social care organisations must ensure policies and procedures are in place to support a culture of openness and transparency when a safety incident has occurred. All health and social care professionals have a professional duty of candour which is overseen by the professional body; the regulator will have in place a process to escalate issues raised.

Health and social care staff have a duty to ensure that clients receive accurate, truthful information about any errors in their care that may lead to harm. Not only should they be informed of the error but this should be accompanied by an apology, which is an expression of sorrow or regret in relation to the incident, as well as support and help to ensure they understand what has happened. An apology is not an admission of guilt but recognition of the responsibility to be open and honest.

When an incident has occurred, you are required to:
- Be open and honest with colleagues, your approved education institution (AEI) and relevant organisations
- Immediately inform your AEI in line with policy so that appropriate support can be provided
- Take part in reviews and investigations, with support from your AEI
- Raise concerns where appropriate
- Refrain from stopping or impeding the raising of concerns.

Case study 1.2

As a health care student or new practitioner, you are working with a team when an untoward incident occurs and a client is harmed. You are not directly involved, but did witness the event.
- Investigate what can be expected of you in this situation
- Identify from your own institution who will provide support to you

Raising concerns (whistleblowing)

Health and social care workers have a duty to raise concerns in relation to poor practice, wrongdoing, illegal activity or where there are risks in an organisation linked to patient safety – for example, unsafe care, unsafe staffing levels, bullying or a poor response to any incident. Any wrongdoing that is covered up, where there is no clear redress or systematic process to examine the issues raised, could result in a public safety issue. Any issue or concern where there is a potential risk to the public, be it from an organisation or an individual, must be raised as a concern.

Raising concerns about wrongdoing or actions within an organisation is commonly known as 'whistleblowing'. People who raise concerns are protected by the Public Interest Disclosure Act (1998). Furthermore, *The Freedom to Speak Up: Raising Concerns* policy for the NHS (April 2016) states that every NHS worker and student has a *professional duty* to report a concern.

Sir Robert Francis QC, in his 2015 report, said that staff needed supportive measures in place to ensure they were free to speak up without fear of recrimination, harassment or bullying. His *Freedom to Speak Up* report (2015) argues that the person raising concerns (the whistleblower) must be protected and requires the organisation to have an open and honest workplace culture where an individual can raise concerns and be supported in doing so.

Initially health and social care workers need to be aware of the whistleblowing policy and procedure within their organisation. The policy will identify who they need to contact internally to raise their concerns – for example, their line manager, employer, lead clinician or, in the case of students, their tutor. Where this is not possible, or matters are not resolved, advice and support can be provided by:

- The Freedom to Speak Up Guardian for the organisation (whistleblowing)
- The Whistleblowing Helpline for the NHS and Social Care
- The professional body
- A trade union
- A solicitor
- A charity, such as Public Concern at Work.

If a concern has not been addressed effectively, it may be necessary to escalate your concerns to an external organisation that has the authority to investigate further. For example:

- The Care Quality Commission
- The Health Inspectorate Wales
- Health Improvement Scotland
- NHS England
- NHS Wales
- NHS Scotland.

Where there are concerns or allegations related to an individual practitioner's fitness to practise, guidance on referral of a health or social care practitioner to their regulatory body can be found on that organisation's website.

Case study 1.3

As a student, you are in clinical practice and notice that the area is very short of staff. You are finding the experience very stressful, as you are unable to focus on your learning needs with your educator because you are needed to provide care as part of the team.

This is not a one-off event but has been a consistent problem in the two weeks you have been in the area. Discussing the problem with the clinical lead has not helped.

- Identify an individual within your AEI to whom you can go for support
- Research the raising concerns/whistleblowing policy within the organisation and discuss actioning it with your AEI.

Case study 1.4

As a newly registered professional in your first post, you are surprised at the clinical/professional manager's manner. You have witnessed them talking to other staff in a bullying and derogatory manner; and you have seen staff upset and in tears. There is generally an unpleasant atmosphere in the workplace, with staff often absent. The manager is not approachable and you are feeling unsupported in your new role.

- Identify who you can go to for support within the organisation
- Research the organisation's whistleblowing policy
- Consider how you would keep a record of your concerns.

Case study 1.5

You are mentoring a health care student in clinical practice. The student has been with you for four weeks and is frequently late arriving at the start of the shift. The student's appearance can be unkempt and they appear disinterested and lacking in enthusiasm.

You have fed back your concerns to the student after the first two weeks, but you have not witnessed any improvement in their attitude.

- Identify who, in the AEI, you can go to for support
- Research the fitness to practise policy of the AEI.

Conclusion

To summarise, this chapter has identified the central importance of professional responsibility in order to ensure high standards of health and social care practice and to maintain public confidence. It has described several key elements in achieving this, including how an ethical code (which identifies the standards of personal and professional behaviour expected of a health and social care professional) can provide guidance for practitioners, employers and the public in terms of what constitutes professional behaviour, as well as ensuring that sound ethical principles can be maintained. Further, it has highlighted the fact that the purpose of regulating health and social care professionals is to protect the public and maintain public confidence.

Regulatory bodies are responsible for setting standards for conduct, professional proficiency, maintenance of the professional register and investigation of complaints to ensure that every professional who wishes to enter, or maintain, their registration meets the criteria for fitness to practise. A professional code assists the public, students and professionals in identifying the standards and expectations of their professional body; it also provides the regulator with mechanisms to judge the practitioner's fitness to practise (FTP).

FTP is about having the right skills, knowledge and character to be a safe practitioner and requires the health and social care student and/or professional to demonstrate a duty of candour when required and to raise concerns or whistleblow if necessary. Whilst raising concerns or whistleblowing is not an easy task, as Heléne Donnelly writes in her preface to this book, it is an essential one, and something all health and social care professionals must embrace if professional ethics, registration, fitness to practise and, ultimately, patient safety and quality of care are to be maintained in everyday practice.

Reflective questions

- Can you critically evaluate the benefits or limitations of professional ethics in the practice of your colleagues or within the policies of the settings where you have worked?
- What are the key challenges on the ground for professional bodies and regulators when setting and maintaining key standards for performance and ethics?
- How might you access support in settings where you have worked, when raising and escalating concerns and whistleblowing?

References

Andrews Report (2014). *'Trusted to Care' – An Independent Review of the Princess of Wales Hospital and Neath Port Talbot Hospital at ABMU Health Board.* Cardiff: Welsh Government.

Banks, S. (2012). *Ethics and Values in Social Work.* 4th edn. Basingstoke: Palgrave Macmillan.

Beauchamp T.L. & Childress J.F. (2013). *Principles of Biomedical Ethics.* 7th edn. Oxford: Oxford University.

Care Quality Commission (2015). *Regulation 20: Duty of Candour.* http://www.cqc.org.uk/sites/default/files/20150327_duty_of_candour_guidance_final.pdf (last accessed 23.11.16).

Ellis, P. (2015). *Understanding Ethics for Nursing Students.* London: Sage Publications Limited.

Francis Inquiry (2013). *Report of the Mid Staffordshire NHS Trust Public Inquiry.* London: The Stationery Office.

Francis, R. (2015). *Freedom to Speak Up.* London: The Stationery Office.

Health Act (1999). London: The Stationery Office.

Health and Care Professions Council (2016). *Standards of Conduct, Performance and Ethics.* London: Health and Care Professions Council.

Health and Care Professions Order (2015). London: The Stationery Office.

Hughes, R.G. (2008). *Patient Safety and Quality: An Evidence Based Handbook for Nurses.* Rockville, MD: Agency for H/C Research and Quality.

Melia, K. (2014). *Ethics for Nursing and Healthcare Practice.* London: Sage Publications Limited.

Morecambe Bay Investigation (2015). *Report of the Morecambe Bay Investigation.* London: The Stationery Office.

NHS England (2016). *Freedom to Speak up: Raising Concerns (Whistleblowing) Policy for the NHS.* London: NHS Improvement NHS England.

Nightingale, F. (1863). *Notes on Hospitals.* London: Longman, Green, Longman, Roberts and Green.

Nightingale, F. (1869). *Notes on Nursing: What it is and What it is not.* London: Dover Publications.

Nursing and Midwifery Council (2010). *Standards for Pre-registration Nursing Education.* London: Nursing and Midwifery Council.

Nursing and Midwifery Council (2015). *The Code: Professional Standards of Practice and Behaviour for Nurses and Midwives.* London: Nursing and Midwifery Council.

Nursing and Midwifery Order (2001). London: The Stationery Office.

Public Interest Disclosure Act. (1998). London: The Stationery Office.

Seedhouse, D. (2009). *Ethics: The Heart of Health Care.* London: John Wiley and Sons Limited.

Skills for Care (2013). *Code of Conduct for Healthcare Support Workers and Adult Social Care Workers in England.* Leeds: Skills for Care and Skills for Health.

The Policy, Ethics and Human Rights Committee (2012). *The Code of Ethics for Social Work: Statement of Principles.* Birmingham: The British Association of Social Work.

Winterbourne View (2012). *Department of Health Review and Response.* London: Department of Health.

World Health Organisation (2011). *Ethics.* http://www.who.int/topics/ethics/en/ (last accessed 23.11.2016).

Chapter 2
Being professional

Janet Kelly and Jacqui Thornton

Learning outcomes
By the end of this chapter you should be able to evaluate:
- Professional behaviours in health and social care settings
- A range of views on how to act professionally for the benefit of people using health and social care services
- Some of the challenges encountered by student practitioners, newly qualified staff and educational institutions when working to fulfil professional expectations in the workforce.

Introduction

When discussing professionalism in health and social care, we have much to learn from commercial enterprises such as John Lewis, with its emphasis on employee partnership. John Lewis enjoys success that comes from the development of a shared workplace culture that supports its partners at all levels in carrying out their professional roles. Central to this vision is the way staff behave towards their colleagues and customers. Being professional in the way you go about your practice enhances the reputation of your professional group and the wider service.

At times, the journey towards becoming a professional can present challenges. Demonstrating the attitudes and behaviours expected by health and social care employers can place very different demands on students from the academic expectations of a university course. Although academic courses mainly focus on theoretical knowledge and technical expertise, students and new graduates are expected to meet the same standards as experienced professionals in the workplace. They may enter a practice environment without considering some of the challenges that lie ahead regarding expectations of them as professionals. This may not only involve applying their knowledge in practice, but may also require them to be professional in how they present themselves in their work, how they go about their business, even how they dress.

Although many areas of our working culture and social interactions have changed in the twenty-first century (along with accelerating technical advances), such issues can have a surprising potential to raise concern about levels of professionalism in staff members, regardless of how technically good they might be within their role. The whole issue of professionalism, professional behaviour and being a professional has challenged students, educators, practitioners and managers for many years and it is essential to consider these matters, especially when transitioning from student life into professional practice.

What is meant by professional behaviour?

Becoming a registered 'professional' does not automatically ensure that an individual is fully aware of the kind of demeanour, behaviour or attitudes that are likely to facilitate the trust and confidence of the public. Professional behaviour is not about a set of rules but relies on an understanding of how to behave in different situations and how to adapt behaviour to be contextually appropriate. It is therefore not solely the role of managers to set standards for professional behaviour. What is needed, instead, is an environment or working culture where all professionals are prepared to regulate and adjust their own behaviour in a complex range of situations. This is partly in order to provide feedback on the behaviour of others, especially when it is judged to be in the best interests of patients/ service users or the reputation of the profession or organisation. It is interesting to reflect on which aspects of behaviour make someone a professional in the eyes of others and how conscious each of us needs to be, when working in health and social care, to ensure that we meet the expectations of our service users and colleagues.

Being a professional means having a job that requires special education, training, or skill; and being professional involves using a wide range of skills and qualities. It is essential for well-regarded and experienced practitioners to model what it means to be professional when supporting students and new graduates to value and develop professional behaviours (Asghari *et al.* 2011).

At times students are challenged in unexpected ways by a placement where their learning needs have to fit around an environment with an emphasis on delivering efficient and effective care for patients or service users. Some may not have worked in a health or social care environment before or been in a situation where their behaviour is carefully monitored and assessed to meet a range of criteria and expectations. For some, working with colleagues or within a system that has very different expectations or values from their peers (especially about communication and professional behaviour) can be stressful or even difficult.

Placements provide students with an ideal opportunity to explore their own values and behaviours as well as learning how to develop a professional demeanour that 'fits' well with the services they are delivering. As part of this process, it is incumbent on professions and organisations to have a clear understanding and be able to articulate the standards of behaviour that they expect within the workplace. This ensures that expectations are clear for learners and new employees in that workplace. Established guides to ethical behaviour for health and social care professionals, such as *The Code* (Nursing and Midwifery Council (NMC) 2015), should be familiar to even the newest students as well as all registered professionals. Such codes stress the need for professional behaviour at all times, although these skills are often acquired through a process of acclimatisation, gathering feedback, reflection and evaluation of each individual's own performance in the work setting (for more on this, see Chapter 3).

Stereotypes should be treated with caution but they have always been prevalent between the generations. Current literature in this area would suggest that a group of 'Millennials' or 'Generation Y' (born between 1980 and 2000) are emerging into the workforce. Whilst members of this generation are seen as techno-savvy and creative thinkers, some are also thought to be overly confident, easily bored and struggle at times to see beyond their own needs. Hills *et al.* (2012) even go as far as to say that 'Generation Y' can be a cause for concern in respect of 'casual communication, poor professional behaviour, shallow professional reasoning and difficulty receiving negative feedback' (p.156). It is certainly true that some students and newer practitioners require clarification about the professional behaviour expected of them from their managers, although, of course, some would say this has always been the case.

It is sometimes suggested that 'professionalism' is conceptually unclear and too vague as a descriptor and therefore unhelpful in the drive to improve professional behaviour in the workplace (Burford *et al.* 2014). An example highlighted by Cuesta-Briand *et al.* (2014) showed that medical students in Australia felt more connected to the notion of 'good doctor' and its associated attributes, whilst they perceived professionalism as an external and imposed construct. Practitioners should therefore be supported to develop specific skills, including the ability to identify appropriate professional behaviour and to engage in open and honest reflection, individually, in teams and within the safe environment of supervision. Student placements and rotational schemes for newer practitioners provide opportunities to test out and practise the skills needed to be a 'good' professional. Whilst this is helpful, there should also be an implicit onus on individuals to espouse professionalism and accountability, and understand the consequences that can follow unprofessional behaviour. Regulators of health and social care professions, such as the NMC (2015) and Health and Care

Professions Council (HCPC 2016a), argue that everyone who makes up the professional workforce, including students, has a duty to do so.

Professionals at all levels of experience can still behave unprofessionally, despite the existence of guidance and policies on professionalism from organisations, the professions themselves and regulators. Examples of cases where professionals have been struck off as a consequence of unprofessional behaviour can be seen on the Health and Care Professions Council Tribunal Service (HCPCTS) website (HCPCTS 2017). So why do some people behave unprofessionally in the workplace, whilst others do not? Is a sense of professionalism inherent or can it be learnt? Where are the demarcations that separate positive and poor professional behaviour and is it the responsibility of the organisation, the profession or the individual to make these distinctions clear?

There are significant consequences if people breach professional behaviour standards and those seen by regulators like the NMC, General Medical Council (GMC) and HCPC are often extreme cases. For instance, having an inappropriate relationship with a service user or verbally assaulting a colleague are likely to lead to enforcement of the conduct policy within the relevant organisation and may result in dismissal from the service and potential removal from the professional register. These occurrences tend to be relatively rare but it is worth noting that such situations often arise when a practitioner's general behaviour has given cause for concern over a longer period. Furthermore, professional behaviour does not have to be extremely poor to hold a person back in their career. For instance, practitioners who display slightly unprofessional behaviour may simply miss out on development opportunities or fail to gain promotion because they do not conduct themselves in a way that is seen to promote the values and characteristics needed for more demanding roles within their profession. On the other hand, practitioners who display positive professional attitudes and behaviour are much more likely to become involved in service development and quality improvements within the workplace and are more likely to report errors and under-performance by their colleagues (Lombarts *et al.* 2014). Supervision and annual appraisal are key workplace support mechanisms for practitioners to gain feedback on their professional behaviour and its impact, and the more an employee can engage in these opportunities, the more they are likely to gain from them.

Personal behaviour – accountability and responsibility

Central to this whole debate about professional behaviour is the concept of accountability, which demands that all professionals are responsible and answerable for their own actions. The HCPC standards of conduct, performance and ethics clarify that 'as a registrant you are personally responsible for the way you behave' (HCPC 2016b, p.4) whilst the NMC states that 'nurses and midwives commit to upholding these standards. This commitment to professional standards is fundamental to being part of a profession' (NMC 2015, p.2). Regulators such as these state that the standards are there to promote and protect the interests of service users and carers. The standards refer to personal and professional behaviour and place the onus on all registrants to ensure 'your conduct justifies the public's trust and confidence in you and your profession' (HCPC 2016b, p.9). The word 'responsible' carries particular weight, making all health and social care professionals morally accountable for their behaviour.

Unfortunately, the conduct of some professionals in the workplace would suggest that they do not sufficiently consider the relevance of personal behaviour to the way they perform in their roles at work. The need to be professional should go without saying but this is not always the case. Being a health or social care professional brings with it a responsibility that perhaps not all new students are aware of when they enrol on their university courses. Organisations like the National Health Service or Social Services have a legal and ethical duty to protect the interests and well-being of their service users.

The ethical and professional codes of conduct of individual professions and regulators also make their members accountable for their behaviour outside the workplace, in situations where their actions may be witnessed by colleagues, employers, services users and/or members of the public (see Chapter 1 and Chapter 7). This is also reinforced in the HCPC (2016a) *Guidance on conduct and ethics for students* and the NMC's statement that their code is to enable students to understand the requirements for qualified nurses and midwives (NMC 2015). These professional codes underline the importance of maintaining certain standards of personal behaviour when undertaking a career in health or social care – a point that may not always be obvious to those beginning a programme of study leading to a professional qualification.

Impact of positive professional behaviour

Research by HCPC (2014) into professionalism highlights positive professional characteristics and values that can be identified across all health and social care professions. The study highlights how essential it is to promote better understanding of the concept of professionalism across professional groups and the fact that professionalism has its basis in individual characteristics and values. The report clarifies the importance of individual professional judgement in the context of a particular situation, and this needs to be reinforced across different professional groups. This links with the authors' own views that the impact of professional behaviour provides a valuable measure of whether the behaviour can be deemed positive or negative and whether there are consequences for the user of the service, the practitioner or the profession.

There is much evidence showing how positive professional behaviour can sustain and improve service delivery (Badri *et al.* 2009, Lombarts *et al.* 2014), and significantly enhance the experience of the users of health and social care services and the outcomes of treatment. This means that practitioners must consider the explicit and implicit messages and motivations of their behaviours in all circumstances in the workplace. For student health or social care professionals, equal importance must be placed on the quality of personal interactions with the users of the service and the quality of the technical intervention provided. Policies such as the *NHS Constitution for England* (Department of Health (DOH) 2015) promote the partnership agenda in provision of care and the importance of good professional relationships.

One of the key characteristics of a practitioner who behaves professionally is self-awareness and this seems to be a crucial quality in people who display highly professional behaviour. They are able to analyse and reflect on their own behaviour, recognising when it has a positive (or, indeed, negative) effect on patient care and team relationships, and taking action as appropriate to the situation. Health and social care professionals and students do not, generally, deliberately intend to behave in a negative way and may be unaware of the impact of their behaviour.

One example is the way some people may struggle to hide boredom or lack of attention; consider perhaps an individual who texts on their mobile or stares out of the window during formal meetings. When challenged, most will admit to drifting off, but they may well be shocked that their behaviour is so obvious to the rest of the group. They may also be surprised to discover that this behaviour is likely to have consequences for them and the profession they represent. Some people might decide to challenge this type of feedback but try putting yourself in a supervisor or practice mentor's position: if you had a mentee who disagreed with all aspects of the developmental feedback you gave them, how confident would you feel about them as a practitioner?

The importance of good communication

Communication style is a key aspect of positive professional behaviour. To ensure that you are seen as a trustworthy health or social care professional, you should incorporate reliability, openness, competence and concern in your communications. Simple things, such as introducing yourself, are very powerful ways of making patients feel valued, as shown by the 'Hello My Name Is …' campaign (NHS England 2015). Likewise, ensuring that the service user's preferred name is used and clarifying the purpose and extent of a contact with an individual can help promote a professional image. The use of diminutives such as 'dear', 'sweetie' or 'babe', whilst seen by some professionals in the past as demonstrating care and warmth, is now widely recognised as undermining dignity (see Chapter 11). *Delivering Dignity* (Commission on Dignity in Care 2012, p.10) highlights the importance of treating people with respect and how individuals who are not supported to maintain their dignity and identity can experience deterioration in skills and self-confidence with subsequent poorer health. Interestingly, in these situations these individuals also tended to display less cooperative and more aggressive responses to care (Williams & Herman 2012).

Whilst these findings are specific to older people, the messages are valuable for the delivery of health or social care for *all* practitioners and underline the way seemingly innocuous professional behaviour can have a widespread impact on well-being. Professionals should ask themselves how the language they use and the way that they communicate affect the people they are working with and the way they are viewed as a professional. Students and new practitioners will need to consider how they promote professionalism within workplace settings where the culture can reinforce acceptance of less professional behaviour.

Most organisations will have policies in place that support practitioners to challenge any behaviour that is not in the best interests of patient care. It is important to remember that this has been learned from defining moments in the history of public service, such as the example at Mid Staffordshire Hospital highlighted by Donnelly in the Preface to this book. Making such a challenge will inevitably be stressful for the practitioner concerned. However, the standards of conduct performance and ethics are clear that the safety and well-being of service users 'always comes before any professional or other loyalties' (HCPC 2016b, p.8) and practitioners must put 'the interests of patients and service users first' (NMC 2015, p.3).

Does appearance matter?

What role does appearance play in this whole debate about professionalism? The *All Wales NHS Dress Code* (NHS Wales 2010, p.7) states that 'patients generally prefer to be treated by staff with tidy hair and a neat appearance and that providing a professional image will promote public confidence'. It further states that 'securing the confidence of the public is paramount in delivering exemplary health care services' (p.2). Evidence has shown that the public is concerned about a number of issues relating to the wearing of NHS uniforms and the behaviour of NHS staff. How potentially controversial is it in this day and age to accept that 'people may use general appearance as a proxy measure of competence and professional practice'? (NHS Wales 2010, p.6). The notion of sacrificing your freedom as an individual when you 'switch on your professionalism' (Finn *et al.* 2010, p.819) is an important concept when considering personal presentation. Whilst personal appearance may be a way of expressing one's identity, wise professionals will ensure that nothing they do regarding their own self-presentation perpetuates any notion of disadvantage for their clients. It is interesting to note that the HCPC *Guidance on conduct and ethics for students* also picks up this theme, explaining that students are required to dress appropriately for placement settings (HCPC 2012).

Respect as a core value of good professionals

Inherent within the actions of practitioners who behave professionally is that they demonstrate universal respect for service users, colleagues, managers and the general public (DOH 2015). This essential element of professional behaviour has a profound impact on the reputation of individual practitioners and on the profession they represent. In clinical situations, demonstrating respect for service users influences their willingness to work collaboratively with professionals and increases their confidence that their needs are being prioritised. Practitioners need to give the implicit message that we value the individual and the service we are offering them. Imagine a situation where you discuss an intervention with an individual and then fail to follow through on your commitment to them. This may create a negative situation in which they may feel they are unimportant, you are not bothered, maybe that you are not committed to their care, they have a lower priority than your other workload issues or perhaps that the intervention was of little value anyway. In this way, the messages professionals give through our behaviour, even subtle ones, have a wider impact on how we and our profession are perceived within the workplace.

One key question is whether professional behaviour is an indicator of practice quality. In other words, is someone who shows low levels of professionalism in their behaviour necessarily a weaker professional practitioner? In universities it is important to develop knowledge and skills to deliver during clinical practice and placements. Professional behaviour is of course considered in universities, but it can be linked to engagement in the academic curriculum or endangering the reputation of the university. This subject might only be considered to relate to the social aspects of the student's life, unless practice settings alert the institution about issues encountered within services hosting placements. The explicit link between professional behaviour and professional practice is most likely to be keenly observed and measured on placement where relationships are more intense and students and their supervisors/mentors are often engaged on a 1:1 basis.

Whilst all universities have 'fitness to practise' processes to examine and sometimes impose sanctions for unprofessional student behaviour amongst health and social care students, these only consider actual behaviour on placement once the student has left the academic environment and gone into real-life service settings (see Chapter 1).

To help raise awareness of practice requirements and professionalism, most universities cover issues related to becoming a professional, especially in the early stages of study programmes. However, this essential aspect of pre-registration courses needs to be further developed, particularly for those students who struggle with it. If even more emphasis was placed on the positive professional behaviours that are considered important for a 'good' professional, this would certainly affect the evaluation of the clinical/practice capabilities of some individuals. These aspects of professional behaviour (for example, good timekeeping, attention to detail, commitment to improvement and being receptive to feedback) are all indicators that these individuals are committed to quality and development and can work effectively in teams. On the other hand, if an individual is always late for work, enthusiastic but lacking in consistency and appears to have difficulty responding to developmental feedback, they may be perceived as not having characteristics that lend themselves to being a thoughtful, self-regulating professional.

Whose judgement is it anyway?

It is highly unlikely that everyone judges professional behaviour in the same way, so whose judgement is most important? The views of service users are crucial but it can be difficult to get honest feedback from service users because they may not wish to express an opinion about a particular professional. Colleagues within one's own profession may have differing personal standards of professional behaviour and may disagree with each other. Similarly, other professions may have specific aspects of performance that they value more or less, which can lead to conflicting messages about what is most important in relation to professional behaviour. Managers may be more concerned about organisational image and the impact of individual performance on the reputation of the department or service. In truth, the perspectives of all of these individuals matter and their views should be actively sought when considering your own professional behaviour, as each will have relevance and will help you understand the potential impact of your behaviour both now and in the future. Services often remember students and practitioners who have a positive professional impact but they equally remember those whose behaviour did not meet expected standards.

Table 2.1 consists of a series of questions that can be used to promote self-reflection on your own behaviour and the way you promote a professional image. These questions may also be used when asking other people to review your performance and comment on aspects of your professional behaviour.

Table 2.1 Self-reflection questions on professional behaviour

Question	Prompts/Ideas
Do I show respect for others? (includes service users/ colleagues/families/ others)	• How am I sensitive to others' needs? • Do I pay attention to the feelings and behaviours of others and make appropriate responses to them? • Does my verbal and non-verbal communication show that I am listening and responding to the needs of the person with whom I am communicating? • Is my respect given, regardless of whether or not I feel the person deserves it? • Do I consider the impact of my decisions on others? • How do I show that I am considering the impact of my behaviour on others?
Am I trustworthy and dependable?	• Do I consistently turn up to work/meetings/appointments on time? • If I have a task to do, is it completed without anyone needing to prompt me about it? • Do I notice when people need my help and respond accordingly? • Am I loyal to my colleagues at all times? • Do I complete tasks consistently or do I just do the ones that I am interested in? • Do I take responsibility for my own work, consistently manage my own work and time, and (if things go wrong) take responsibility for the things I haven't done well?
Am I a person who maintains confidentiality in and out of work?	• Do I ensure that I am careful about where and with whom I hold conversations about service users or colleagues? • Do I ever talk about service users or colleagues at home or in public in such a way that their identity could be revealed? (including via social media)? • Do I ensure that I am open with service users about the meaning of confidentiality?
How well do I present a professional image?	• Do I ever wear things that suggest I am not serious about my work role? • Is my dress and presentation acceptable to the service users, colleagues and other staff with whom I work? • What image does the language I use and my non-verbal communication convey to the people with whom I work? • Does this communication indicate that I am serious about them and the work that I do? • Do I represent my profession well – for example, if an individual had only ever had contact with me, would they have a good impression of my profession?
Are my work relationships appropriate?	• Do I ensure that my relationships are always clear and can't be misunderstood by the people with whom I work? • Could my relationships with service users and colleagues be misconstrued by others?

	• Do my work relationships sometimes cause me to behave in a way that makes me feel uncomfortable, e.g. being late because of others/taking part in inappropriate conversations/ breaking rules? • Do I work collaboratively with others? • Do I sometimes allow others to do the work or take over and not allow people to contribute?
Do I ever behave unprofessionally?	• Do people ever comment on my behaviour or does their non-verbal communication suggest that they are uncomfortable with the way I behave? • Do I ever behave in a way that would be embarrassing if my manager/ supervisor saw me? • Do I act differently when I am with certain groups of people? • Do I sometimes feel that I have let myself and the service down? • Am I sometimes angry or moody at work and show this in the way I behave? • If I am not happy with aspects of the service, do I complain to others but not offer ways to improve the situation? • When outside of work, do I still consider that I need to act in a way that does not compromise my professional role? This includes when I am socialising, in my personal life and when using social networking sites. • Is my use of social media compromising my professional image? • Would I be happy for my employer or service users to see what is posted online about me or by me?
Do I demonstrate initiative and commitment to my work?	• How do I demonstrate that I am generating ideas to improve my practice? • How do I follow through these ideas into actions that improve practice and service delivery? • Who do I work with to do this? • Do I wait for my manager/ supervisor to give me things to do, rather than taking the initiative in finding work and new projects? • Do I sometimes complain that others get more opportunities that I do? • Do I take supervision seriously, demonstrating that I am striving for excellence and continued development of skills, attitudes and knowledge? • How do I encourage and support those with whom I work to develop and improve the quality of their practice?

Conclusion

The issue of professional behaviour is extremely important in any discussion about what makes a successful practitioner in health and social care. Appraising professional behaviour can become difficult or contentious if viewed as a judgemental 'right' or 'wrong'. However, if it is viewed as a continuum, with each practitioner taking personal responsibility for the way they conduct themselves in the workplace, it provides a more helpful starting point for any individual undertaking a career in a health or social care profession. Personal reflection is crucial if practitioners are to understand the impact that their demeanour (behaviour and appearance) has on their overall professional performance and how that is perceived.

Most organisational policies specify what is generally acceptable and unacceptable in terms of conduct and presentation. All employees of those organisations are obliged (through their contract of employment) to adhere to the guidelines that have been laid down. Apart from that, it is incumbent on students and new graduates to use more experienced practitioners as role models for appropriate professional behaviour and to use reflection as a tool to seriously consider how they go about their role and how this helps or hinders the therapeutic goals of their client groups. By the same token, it is incumbent on all qualified professionals to model positive behaviour in the workplace (Asghari *et al.* 2011, NMC and CNOs 2017) and to create environments that enable open and honest reflection on professional behaviour.

It would seem sensible that professional behaviour should continue to be emphasised in university courses, providing students with the opportunity to explore this complex issue and develop appropriate skills before they go on placement and graduate into the workplace. It may be helpful for universities to implement this in collaboration with local service managers and senior practitioners.

Now you have read this chapter, you are now advised to think about the highest levels of professional behaviour you have seen or read about in day-to-day practice for your particular discipline. Use the questions in Table 2.1 to prompt your thinking.

Reflective questions

- Choose a situation from your practice where you think that your professional behaviour, or that of a colleague, has made a real difference to a service user – what was it that worked so well and why?
- What can you do or change to become a highly regarded role model for those around you?

References

Asghari, F., Fard. N.N. & Atabaki. A. (2011). Are we proper role models for students? Interns' perception of faculty and residents' professional behaviour. *Postgraduate Medical Journal.* **87** (1030), 519–23.

Badri, M., Attia, S. & Ustadi, A. (2009). Healthcare quality and moderators of patient satisfaction: testing for causality. *International Journal of Health Care Quality Assurance.* **22** (4), 382–410.

Burford, B., Morrow, G., Rothwell, C. & Illing, J. (2014). Professionalism education should reflect reality: findings from three health professions. *Medical Education.* **48** (4), 361–74.

Commission on Dignity in Care. (2012). *Delivering Dignity: Securing dignity in care for older people in hospitals and care homes.* http://www.nhsconfed.org/~/media/Confederation/Files/Publications/Documents/Delivering_Dignity_final_report150612.pdf. (last accessed 18.12.2016).

Cuesta-Briand, B., Auret, K., Johnson, P. & Playford, D. (2014). 'A world of difference': a qualitative study of medical students' views on professionalism and the 'good doctor'. *BMC Medical Education.* **14** (77).

Department of Health (2015). *The NHS Constitution for England.* https://www.gov.uk/government/uploads/system/uploads/attachment_data/file/480482/NHS_Constitution_WEB.pdf (last accessed 18.12.2016).

Finn, G., Garner, J. & Sawdon, M. (2010). 'You're judged all the time!' Students' views on professionalism: a multi-centre study. *Medical Education.* **44** (8), 814–25.

Health and Care Profession Council Tribunal Service. (2017). *Hearings and Decisions. Recent Decisions.* https://www.hcpts-uk.org/hearings/recentdecisions (last accessed 27.04.2017).

Health and Care Profession Council (HCPC) (2016a). *Guidance on conduct and ethics for students.* London: HCPC.

Health and Care Profession Council. (2016b). *Standards of conduct, performance and ethics.* London: HCPC.

Health and Care Professions Council (HCPC) (2014). *Professionalism in Healthcare Professionals: Research report.* http://www.hcpc-uk.org/assets/documents/10003771Professionalisminhealthcareprofessionals.pdf (last accessed 19.12.2016).

Health and Care Profession Council (HCPC) (2012). *Guidance on conduct and ethics for students.* London: HCPC.

Hills, C., Rhan, S., Smith. D.R. & Warren-Forward, H. (2012). The impact of 'Generation Y' occupational therapy students on practice education. *Australian Occupational Therapy Journal.* **59** (2),156–63.

Lombarts, K.M., Plochg, T., Thompson, C.A., Arah, O.A. and on behalf of the DUQuE Project Consortium. (2014). Measuring Professionalism On Medicine and Nursing: results of a European survey. *PLOS ONE.* **9** (5), e97069. https://www.ncbi.nlm.nih.gov/pmc/articles/PMC4029578/ (last accessed 18.12.2016).

National Health Service (NHS) Wales (2010). *All Wales NHS Dress Code. Free to Lead, Free to Care.* http://www.wales.nhs.uk/sitesplus/documents/862/Attachment%20-%20NHS%20Dress%20Code.pdf (last accessed 18.12.2016).

National Health Service England (2015). *Campaign for compassion in care hits a new milestone. NHS England's Chief Nursing Officer (CNO) Jane Cummings has praised the 'Hello My Name Is …' campaign started by terminally ill Dr Kate Granger.* https://www.england.nhs.uk/2015/02/hellomynameis/ (last accessed 18.12.2016).

Nursing and Midwifery Council & Chief Nursing Officers (2017). *Enabling Professionalism in Nursing and Midwifery Practice.* https://www.nmc.org.uk/globalassets/sitedocuments/other-publications/enabling-professionalism.pdf (last accessed 19.05.2017).

Nursing and Midwifery Council (NMC) (2015). *The Code: Professional Standards of Practice and Behaviour for Nurses and Midwives.* London: NMC.

Williams, K. & Herman, R. (2011). Linking resident behavior to dementia care communication: Effects of emotional tone. *Behavior Therapy.* **42** (1), 42–46.

Chapter 3
Professionalism: A journey from novice to expert practitioner

Gary Strong

Learning outcomes

By the end of this chapter you will be able to:

- Evaluate how professional values are learned and shaped, using the 'novice to expert framework' from new student to established professional
- Examine aspects of professional skills, attitudes and thinking that contribute to expectations of professional behaviour as we face the challenges of practice
- Discuss and reflect on examples of competent and expert professional behaviour relating to your own profession.

This chapter will introduce the 'learning journey' of professionalism using theoretical and practical examples, helping you to build your understanding of what it means to develop professional expertise, values and behaviours. You will see how the concept of a 'learning journey' applies as much to your attitudes and ideas as to your knowledge and skills.

Applying to study health and social care

Let's start at the beginning and consider what professionalism might look like at the outset of your 'learning journey'. When you apply to university, you write a personal statement. The academic and professional staff who read that statement want to know if you are capable of developing the attributes of a health or social care professional. Of course, they also want to know if you have the academic ability and commitment to complete the qualification.

At this early stage, they are keen to find evidence indicating that this person has the qualities and values that will enable them to become an expert in caring for others, in the complex, rapidly changing world of twenty-first century health and social care. Your personal statement therefore marks the start of your journey.

You may also notice that your course is subject to *Values Based Recruitment*, an approach to interviewing for staff and students adopted by the NHS to explore the qualities expected from people working in this sector, as embedded in the NHS Constitution (Health Education England 2016). Whether you are a school leaver, or someone with years of work experience about to embark upon a new career, these steps mean you will have been given the opportunity to review your life experiences, reflect upon what you have learned from them and shown how they have prepared you to make the journey ahead. These are your first steps on the road to becoming an expert health or social care practitioner.

Consider the difference between these two personal statements:

> 'I realised that I wanted to become a paramedic when I saw an ambulance stop at a road accident. The paramedics jumped out and were straight onto it. I know now that I want an action-packed career that gives me the chance to help others and save lives. I have joined the Red Cross and learned basic first aid and I cannot wait to learn more medical skills.'

> 'Paramedics make difficult decisions every day, caring for others. Volunteering in a care home for older people has helped me to realise what empathy is: the ability to understand another person's situation and suffering and demonstrate that I care. This can be challenging when you are tired and faced with multiple competing demands, and even more so if you are faced with challenging behaviour by a client. But in order to improve the lives of others I have learned that I must respect them and work hard to give the best service to everyone, whatever their background or problem.'

Neither of these statements is 'wrong', but which one do you think offers the best understanding of the role of a health professional – in this case, a paramedic? Reflect now, why is this?

The five-stage model of skill acquisition

In this chapter, we will map out the journey from novice to expert and illustrate this with an example group of emerging health professionals, although these principles apply just as much when entering practice in social care. The phrase 'novice to expert' was coined by two brothers, Stuart and Hubert Dreyfus. The Dreyfus brothers worked at the University of California in the 1970s and 1980s, devoting their research to understanding the process by which we learn a new skill and eventually become expert at it. They considered four examples: flying an aeroplane, playing chess, driving a car and learning a second language (Dreyfus 2004). These are all complex skills requiring a blend of physical and mental activity.

Stuart Dreyfus (2004) decided that when we learn a new skill, we move through five levels of learning or five measures of our ability to carry out the task. These are:

1. **Novice** – when you are learning a skill for the first time, under instruction, using a basic set of rules

2. **Advanced beginner** – when you have become familiar with the basics of the skill and are learning to adapt some of the rules to a changing environment

3. **Competent** – when you have begun to realise how varied the environment is, and you are starting to make your own judgements about using the skill, with reference to the basic rules

4. **Proficient** – when you are consciously using your knowledge of the rules and your experience to make informed decisions on using the skill

5. **Expert** – when your use of the skill appears intuitive to others, because – based on your knowledge and experience – you are able to deploy it rapidly and effectively in an ever-changing environment.

These are more than abstract ideas and very relevant to gaining expertise in any area. Think about learning to drive a car. As a *novice*, you are told when to change gear, when to brake, when to indicate. A novice must follow the rules to manoeuvre the car safely. That said, rules alone are not enough: you may be told to change up a gear once the car reaches a certain speed, but the first time you drive up a steep hill you will need to modify this behaviour.

You start to figure out for yourself that the change needs to occur later, with a higher engine speed. You are now becoming an *advanced beginner*, no longer simply relying on the rules, but starting to read the road conditions, listen to the sound of the engine and change gear when necessary. You are learning to piece together the different components of the skill of driving, under the guidance and, when necessary, the instructions of an experienced driver.

Taking the next step and becoming *competent* is hard work: you would need an enormous set of rules to cover every possible situation you might encounter when driving a car, and there is no time to look up the rules when you are halfway round a bend. 'In general' comments Dreyfus (2004, p.179), 'if one seeks the safety of rules, one will not get beyond competence'. So you are now integrating knowledge and experience and the first time you drive without an instructor is usually nerve racking.

Over time, you will develop your own library of driving experiences. You will refer to these (sometimes consciously) but you will increasingly develop a well-informed intuition that enables you to negotiate hazards safely with less effort. You are becoming *proficient*. You can now make decisions that keep you safe in a wide variety of driving situations.

By the time you become an *expert*, you will largely be unaware that you are making these decisions – unless you meet a particularly new, challenging situation. You will, in the main, be doing what comes naturally.

Many of the skills we use in health and social care are comparable to the examples cited by Dreyfus in that they require a blend of cognitive (mental) and psychomotor (physical) actions and activities. Consequently, the model is very useful when considering the education of health and social care professionals. Taking an individual's blood pressure, conducting an interview with a client, writing up notes, assessing movement are just a few examples. What can you add to the list from your own chosen profession? As you reflect, you may conclude that a great many of the skills needed by health or social care professionals can be developed in this way.

Now think about what all those who work in health and social care have in common. The understanding and application of professional values are fundamental for all of us. Reflect upon these values in the light of the 'learning journey' described by Dreyfus (2004). When we acquire new learning, we start out as a novice. Then, after a while, we become an 'advanced beginner'. As we practise and refine what we have learned, we become 'competent', then 'proficient', then eventually – if we practise well – an 'expert'. Professional attitudes and behaviours can be learned, developed and refined. Expert professionalism is your goal; and the very nature of expertise for professionals means you will continue on this journey throughout your career. Indeed, one of the reasons that many people are attracted to the health and caring professions is this very need for continuing professional development as new areas of practice emerge and services demand new things from us as they change and evolve (see Chapter 4).

As long ago as 1956, Benjamin Bloom recognised that we learn in three different areas or 'domains': psychomotor, where we learn mechanical skills; cognitive, where we acquire new knowledge; and affective, where we develop and change our attitudes (Bloom *et al.* 1956). Think of the example of taking someone's blood pressure. The skill of applying the cuff is largely psychomotor, requiring hand-eye coordination. To understand what the reading means, we need the cognitive ability to learn the basics of the cardiovascular system. But we also need to gain consent from our patients, make them comfortable in our presence and perhaps also counsel them on the implications of the reading. These are professional skills, learned in the *affective* domain.

For some students, the problem with affective learning and professional values is that it all sounds so abstract. The majority of health and social care students would much rather get on with learning something more tangible. A client who needs assessment or a set of baseline observations somehow seem more 'real' to us. In truth, these and other procedural activities can only be successful if they are embedded in a professional approach to care and the theory/evidence to guide it.

Novices

To illustrate this, let's meet Charlotte, Roger, Andy and Louisa, four health care students sharing accommodation in their first year at university. Charlotte is studying to be an occupational therapist, Roger a nurse, Andy a physiotherapist and Louisa a paramedic. Here is a snippet of their conversation before dinner one evening in their first year:

> *Andy: What are you two up to?*
>
> *Louisa: Taking a selfie! Don't you think we look good in uniform?*
>
> *Roger: An interprofessional selfie, with silly faces!*
>
> *Charlotte: So ... what do you plan to do with it?*
>
> *Roger: Post it, of course! 'Ready to start saving lives' ... or something like that.*
>
> *Andy: You've only just started. What do you know about it?*
>
> *Charlotte: Have you read the placement handbook? There's a section on social media and another on wearing uniform. I really think you should read it before you go any further.*
>
> *Louisa: We were only having a bit of fun. Look at you, you've gone all serious on us.*
>
> *Roger: Charlotte might have a point. I don't want to find we are breaking the rules in our first term.*

As novice professionals, our four flatmates are sharing an important learning experience. They are having a bit of banter together, but in the process they are discovering that their human drives and emotions might lead them into unprofessional territory. What mistakes are they at risk of making, and how can they learn from these mistakes? How do you view their conversation in the light of the standards set out below (Health and Care Professions Council 2016a, p.14)?

- You should be aware that your conduct and behaviour outside your programme may affect whether or not you are allowed to complete your programme or register with us.
- You should not claim that you have knowledge, skills, qualifications and experience which you do not.
- You should be honest about your role with service users, carers and others.

- You should make sure that your personal appearance is appropriate for your practice placement environment.

Charlotte is reminding her flatmates of the rules. They are novices, learning to apply newly discovered regulations to their lives. These are principles that they may well need to read and read again, in order to be sure about the behaviours that are appropriate – and inappropriate – for a learner in health and social care. Andy and Louisa did not deliberately set out to be unprofessional or inappropriate but they have not considered the possible implications of their actions. What may appear to be a harmless 'selfie' could easily appear to others as a misrepresentation of their current role, or lead to inappropriate comment on social media. If seen by a patient or service user, the 'selfie' might undermine confidence or even lead to a complaint. Universities have regulations about the wearing of uniform for good reasons, to protect their students as well as the confidence of service users.

When learning about professional behaviours, we must begin to apply risk assessments to our actions and ask whether we might be unintentionally contravening important principles. Louisa and Roger are still learning to apply these principles to their behaviour and, like all novices, they will need reminding of the 'rules' in order to become more familiar with them and apply them in new situations.

As another example of learning the rules, let's consider how our four flatmates confront the issue of confidentiality.

Andy: Hey Roger, I think I saw one of your mates in the clinic yesterday.

Roger: Oh yes, who was that?

Louisa: Hang on, hang on, you two... Are we talking about a patient here?

Charlotte: We prefer the term 'client'.

Louisa: Patient, client, service user... Whatever we call them, we have to respect confidentiality. A person's health care is their own business and we have no right to talk about it without their consent.

What is going on here should be clear. Louisa has spotted the risk and come to the aid of her friends. She has taken on board the principle of confidentiality and she is taking the opportunity to help others to put this into practice.

Consider this standard (Health and Care Professions Council 2012b, p.7):

You must treat information about service users as confidential. You must only disclose information if you have permission; if the law allows this; if it is in the service user's best interests; or if it is in the public interest, such as it is necessary to protect public safety or prevent harm to other people.

Advanced beginners

We meet our four flatmates again towards the end of their second year. Already now, they have experienced many hours of face-to-face contact with patients, clients or service users. Some of these experiences have been deeply challenging, as they have attempted to apply professional values and standards to their placement experiences. They find themselves together in an interprofessional seminar group, encouraged to discuss some of the difficulties they have faced:

> *Roger: I think the hardest thing for me has been knowing what to do next when I am on a busy ward. Everyone has the same right to good care, don't they, but some folk can be such a pain. While I am deciding between helping one patient to the loo, assisting another to finish eating their lunch and helping a third who has slipped too far down the bed, there is always one who thinks they are entitled to my undivided attention the whole day and keeps finding some random reason to call me over. The very first item on the NMC Code says that I must 'treat people with kindness, respect and compassion' [Nursing and Midwifery Council 2015, p.4], but I do find it hard to give the same level of care to everyone. My mentor supervision is very good, but increasingly she is wanting me to work it out for myself.*

> *Charlotte: Is that like our HCPC standards?*

> *Roger: Yes, I think so. Have a look here, the first section is all about respect and dignity.*

> *Andy: Let's see, let's have a read. Huh! Some of the patients I've been seeing should read this. They don't treat me with respect and dignity. I overheard one the other day in the waiting area... 'I'm seeing that one who always has the gay student with him. I can spot one a mile off, you know.'*

> *Charlotte: Andy, it's us who sign up to these standards, not the clients. When you are caring for people, you are going to get all sorts to deal with. When you think about it, respect and dignity cover just about everything we do. We have to try to be consistent. I've had a few dodgy things said to me when I've been trying to help with a needs assessment, but my mentor has been brilliant with her guidance. A lot of it is about trying to understand why people think and act the way they do and what their real social needs are.*

> *Louisa: I think what I find hardest is when we go back to the same patient on a regular basis. They might have an alcohol problem, or they might be very depressed, or they might just be someone who keeps falling over, but it is so frustrating when nobody has done anything about it since last time, and when they won't listen to you. We are supposed to make shared decisions with them these days, but some people seem to want to make some very bad decisions.*

> *Roger: Advocacy is really important too. Just last week I had to work with a patient who wanted to be discharged to a situation where she was really unable to look after herself. Do I advocate for her safety, or for her autonomy?*

Our four friends are now learning to apply principles of professionalism in a variety of difficult circumstances. Like the car driver navigating new traffic conditions in new places, they know the basic principles of professional behaviour, but each new case brings a different set of parameters within which they must apply these principles. To attain competence, they must continue to work hard at this, and at times it will be emotionally as well as mentally draining. With practice, it will become part of what they normally do.

By now, each of them has professional skills, some of which they can perform with barely a second thought. At the same time they are learning new ones; so, as they attain competence in one skill, they are still novices in another. The pathway to competence in the application of professional values is no different. For example, in their first year, Charlotte, Andy, Louisa and Roger were novices in confidentiality. By and large, this is now embedded in their practice and they are very careful to avoid any possible identifiers in their conversation. They are now advanced beginners, discussing how to maintain their standards in more complex situations. In just over a year's time, they will graduate, and their university will inform their respective regulatory bodies that they meet the standards required to register as professionals in health and social care. This tells the wider world that they are competent professionals.

Competence and independent practice go hand in hand. A practitioner who is not yet competent should not practise without supervision. Registration brings with it the removal of the safety net of supervised practice that is needed for students. Many find this prospect a bit scary, and as we fast-forward to the end of their final year, we find that Roger, Charlotte, Louisa and Andy share the same mixture of excitement and apprehension as any other graduates in health and social care. They all agree that they have enjoyed their discussions of professionalism and professional values, and decide to get together again in a few months' time and compare notes on each other's progress. This is a significant decision.

Benner (1984) noticed that emotional engagement is key to the journey from novice to expert. If you are passionate about your profession and its contribution to health and social care, you will want to keep learning. This does not stop at graduation. Rather, a new chapter begins, in which competence is built upon and proficiency is developed. You are thrust out of one comfort zone, just as it was getting comfortable, and gradually become attuned to a new level of operating. The same complex problems confront you in your practice, but your library of experiences has grown, and so has your ability to select and apply principles and experiences to new situations. It is unlikely that you will notice when you become proficient. In fact this process may continue throughout your career, despite your ever-increasing levels of expertise and skill. It will happen as long as you are willing to keep learning. Consider the conversation that occurs when our four friends next meet.

Competence to proficiency

Roger has set up a closed Facebook group so that they can share a few ideas, including when and where to meet. It takes months to sort out a suitable date, due to their working hours, and when they finally get together it is a year after graduation and they have settled on a camping trip. On a wet afternoon in a quiet country pub, Charlotte reminds them that they have a bit of an agenda:

Charlotte: So we agreed we would do something like that seminar we had in our second year... Pick one really difficult experience and talk about how we dealt with it.

Roger: Can I get another beer first?

Louisa: Only if you go first!

Roger buys them all another drink, then looks around.

Roger: Just making sure no-one is listening in.

Andy: Must be a good one...

Louisa: Look, even before we know Roger's story, think about it, this is one of our problems now. We need to keep reflecting and learning, but everything we deal with is sensitive, confidential. Some of it would be upsetting if we were overheard. It's OK at work. If and when we get a meal break, we pull an incident apart and put it back together again and learn heaps in the process. How do you guys do that?

Charlotte: We use supervision, mainly.

Louisa: We have a clinical supervisor but we only see him if we've done something wrong.

Charlotte: Really? We have monthly meetings.

Andy: We try to, but we are usually too busy.

Roger: We often have informal debriefs in the staff room. This one time, I walked in and one of my colleagues was in tears. Turns out she had given the wrong dose of a sedative to a patient. They had to call the doc to administer a reversal agent. He was not amused, and she thought she was going to lose her job and her registration. I know her pretty well – she started just before me, and I know she really cares about her work. So I went over to chat to her, and gradually the others just left me to it.

Charlotte: What did you say?

Roger: Well, the ward manager had told her to fill in a clinical incident form right away. I knew it had to be done, and I thought it might help her to focus a bit, so I helped her get the facts down. I remembered some of the patient safety stuff we did in our final year, and reminded her that we have to report incidents like this and learn from them, in order to minimise the risk of them happening in future. She kept saying 'they'll sack me', and I kept saying 'no they won't, you were honest about your mistake'. I looked up the Trust policy on incident reporting and it was all about root cause analysis. It said something like, 'we do not seek to punish, we seek to learn and improve'. By this time she had used nearly a box of tissues, but I think she began to feel more positive.

Andy: What did the Trust do?

Roger: They interviewed her, and I went along to support her. They were pretty cool about it all and thanked her for her honesty. In the end, it turned out that this was one of several drug errors over a couple of months. Not long afterwards, they introduced a whole new checking procedure on the wards. My friend got an informal warning and we all had to do an online course on drug safety.

In this brief story, Roger has demonstrated a high level of professional competence. He has supported a colleague at a difficult time, whilst at the same time acknowledging and understanding that the safety of patients is paramount. His behaviour embodies some important principles and standards. Under the heading 'work co-operatively', the Nursing and Midwifery Council Code (2015, p.8) states that nurses and midwives must:

- work with colleagues to preserve the safety of those receiving care
- share information to identify and reduce risk
- be supportive of colleagues who are encountering health or performance problems. However, this support must never compromise or be at the expense of patient or public safety.

This was the first time Roger had had to focus his professional values on an issue like this. He checked the rules, and mentally checked some of his learning from university. He knew he needed to look after the safety of the patient and the welfare of his colleague, although his concerns perhaps surfaced in a different order. The experience of synthesising important professional concepts should give him confidence in his ability to think and act professionally. On that wet afternoon in the pub, his friends are impressed, and tell him so.

After a year or two of growing competence in professional practice in health and social care, it is likely that some or all of our four friends will be considered ready to help new staff in their transition to practice. Looking after and supporting a new entrant to your profession is a challenging and demanding role; and, whether you are classed as a preceptor, a mentor, a practice educator, or whatever terminology your profession uses, you will need to have demonstrated proficiency in your practice.

Dreyfus (2004, p.179) states that 'the proficient performer, after spontaneously seeing the point and the important aspects of the current situation, must still decide what to do. And to decide, he or she must fall back on detached rule and maxim following.' This theoretical statement sheds light on Roger's actions in the situation he described. If he thinks and acts like this regularly, checking and abiding by his professional standards, then he is a 'proficient professional'. The more he does it, the larger his library of experiences grows, each one turning theory into practice. He is not yet an expert, but he is ready to take on the role of supporting a new professional on the same journey. The Department of Health (2010, p.17) states that the attributes of a preceptor may take up to two years to develop. They include 'being an effective and inspirational role model and demonstrating professional values, attitude and behaviours'.

Proficiency to expertise

Let's fast-forward again to another get-together, organised by Charlotte and Roger. Busy with their careers and families, they have again struggled to find time to meet, and they are shocked to discover that they have now spent almost as long in practice as they did at university!

Louisa: Are you guys looking after students now?

Charlotte: Not yet. I've been putting it off, but I'm getting one soon, I think.

Roger: I haven't done the mentoring course yet.

Andy: I've been co-mentoring with one of my colleagues who is a bit more experienced. I really enjoy passing on what I've learned. Luckily, we have a good student. There are some daft ones!

Louisa: There are... but then, that was us a few years ago, wasn't it? I've taken on a student, and all she wants to talk about is road accidents, but I've had to help her a lot with confidentiality and communication. The first day she was out with me, I wanted to confiscate her phone! I think she is now starting to understand why.

Charlotte: I must admit, I've looked at one or two students and listened to the things they say, and recognised the old Charlotte from a few years ago.

Andy: What you realise after a while, and it's a bit scary, is that they are watching you and learning from you like some kind of expert.

Louisa: Yes. To them, we are now the experts.

None of our four friends would consider themselves to be experts. But they have worked hard at developing expertise. Ericsson *et al.* (1993) argue that the differences between expert performers and normal adults reflect a lifetime of deliberate effort to improve performance in a particular area.

The ideas of Ericsson *et al.* (1993) have largely influenced activities such as sport and music. But the old adage 'practice makes perfect' applies equally to professional behaviour.

So how can we define an expert professional? In Dreyfus' terms, 'among many situations, all seen as similar with respect to plan or perspective, the expert has learned to distinguish those situations requiring one reaction from those demanding another' (Dreyfus 2004, p.180). For Charlotte, Roger, Louisa and Andy, their journey of professionalism has led them to a point where they behave decisively, and often instinctively follow the patterns and principles expected of a health care professional. They act consistently in the best interests of service users, they uphold the reputation of their professions and, in doing so, they have become role models to the professionals of the future. A new stage in their journey has begun, and that is where we must leave them.

Conclusion

What have we learned in this chapter? Professionalism comprises a complex set of skills that apply in multiple ever-changing situations. Like any other skills, they can be learned using a basic set of rules. They can then be practised and applied until competence, then proficiency, is reached, and the skills become part of our day-to-day professional practice. These skills become more complex over time, from early student studies to the skill levels required by expert practitioners.

We have considered just a few of the many situations in which the 'rules' of professionalism must be applied to fulfil the obligations and expectations of professional behaviour. You should be able to understand professional principles and practise professional behaviours. The examples of Charlotte, Roger, Louisa and Andy are presented to show how professionals can discuss and reflect upon what we are learning in each new situation, irrespective of our chosen profession. By doing this, you too can set out on the road to developing your own professional expertise whatever challenges you may face.

Reflective questions

- In your own health or social care profession, what aspects of professional skills, attitudes and thinking make someone either appear competent or stand out as more expert?
- What are the key influences in helping you learn about your own professional values and informing your professional behaviour? How can you optimise these in practice or when reflecting on your professional behaviour?
- How might these influences change as you move forward in your career facing the complex challenges of more specialised or managerially orientated practice?

References

Benner, P. (1984). *From novice to expert: Excellence and power in clinical nursing practice*. Menlo Park, California: Addison-Wesley.

Bloom, B., Engelhart, M.D., Furst, E.J., Hill, W.H. & Krathwohl, D.R. (1956). *Taxonomy of educational objectives: Handbook I, The cognitive domain*. New York: Longman.

Department of Health (2010). *Preceptorship Framework for Newly Registered Nurses, Midwives and Allied Health Professionals*. London: Department of Health.

Dreyfus, S.E. (2004). The five-stage model of adult skill acquisition. *Bulletin of Science Technology and Society*. **24** (3), 177–81.

Ericsson, K.A., Krampe, R.T. & Tesch-Romer, C. (1993). The role of deliberate practice in the acquisition of expert performance. *Psychological Review*. **100** (3), 363–406.

Health and Care Professions Council (2016a). *Guidance on Conduct, and Ethics for Students*. London: Health and Care Professions Council.

Health and Care Professions Council (2016b). *Standards of Conduct, Performance and Ethics*. London: Health and Care Professions Council.

Health Education England (2016). *Values based recruitment*. https://www.hee.nhs.uk/our-work/attracting-recruiting/values-based-recruitment (last accessed 9.4.2017).

Nursing and Midwifery Council (2015). *The Code: Professional standards of practice and behaviour for nurses and midwives*. London: Nursing and Midwifery Council.

Chapter 4

Embracing professionalism: Becoming a responsible autonomous practitioner

Lyn Westcott

Learning outcomes
By the end of this chapter you will be able to understand:
- The characteristics, skills and experiences that contribute to becoming and remaining a responsible autonomous practitioner
- The factors that build and maintain responsible, thoughtful and autonomous practitioners, including their role and influence within pre-registration education and professional practice
- How to ensure that practitioners continue to remain responsible and developing professionals, despite working in challenging and ever-changing environments.

Introduction
The vital personal transition from student to professional practitioner involves becoming responsible and autonomous. This typically involves discovering, acquiring, using and refining both professional knowledge and skills. In this way, a potential practitioner prepares for their working life by growing a baseline of knowledge year by year during pre-registration education to become ready for their career, which – for the youngest of graduates – could now be well over 40 years long!

During their working life, practitioners build on this baseline, possibly choosing to specialise and broaden their skill set to include greater leadership and management of their service. Accepting a role as a professional means accepting that knowledge will not stay still. Instead, there is an expectation of ever-growing skills and expert judgement or wisdom and the professional is expected to be an active agent of change and their own development. This is not only a personal journey but one in which these expectations are encouraged through career development that is guided and regulated by organisations that have an interest either in the professions (professional bodies) or protecting people who use the services (regulatory bodies guided by statute). So far, so good, but how does this all happen and why is it so important for health and social care professionals and those who use their services?

To explore this process, we will consider the characteristics, skills and experiences that contribute to a person becoming and remaining a responsible, autonomous practitioner and will think about why this is so important. You will be challenged to consider how these areas can apply to a range of professional practice environments, including working in more isolated posts. A number of themes will be discussed, which can make responsible practice easier or more difficult, including how to engage in opportunities and work around processes.

This chapter will also discuss those important personal resources that can really help practitioners ensure they have fulfilling careers, with a focus on resilience and accommodating change which can challenge morale and, for some people, may seem overwhelming. We will also consider aspects of career development linked to being a responsible contemporary practitioner and the challenges this may bring at a personal level. Finally, the professional responsibility to become and remain a responsible autonomous practitioner will be considered throughout the discussion.

Professional qualification and continuing professional development (CPD): a guided journey

When someone decides to become a health or social care professional, they experience a unique personal journey in making that decision. They may be inspired by the care and service given to a close family member, or they may discover an interest in the profession through careers advice. Alternatively, they may see a professional at work or, perhaps, come across something on social media that inspires them to apply to a programme of study. This begins a voyage of discovery, marked by a growth of knowledge and skill that needs to continue throughout their career. They may have a personal drive that motivates them to develop greater expertise or they may be responding to advances in service delivery, or new knowledge that guides professional practice or societal change.

As soon as they apply for a place to study, the student practitioner will be guided through a series of progressively complex demands, in academic and real practice situations. This process aims to increase knowledge and sharpen professional thinking and reasoning, whilst enhancing both competence and confidence when carrying out sets of unique and specialised tasks. Success in a programme leading to a qualification provides clear evidence that the learner has completed an important passage to become fit for professional practice. This marks the beginning of a career role where expectations will include being both responsible and confident when undertaking whatever scope of professional practice the job requires, and also demonstrating consistent competency.

Whilst completion of any initial pre-registration education is a significant landmark for a health or social care professional, expectations of the new practitioner's achievements to that point will have been determined by a wide range of stakeholders. The educational institution (in the UK, usually a university) will have academic standards expected to achieve certificates, diplomas and degrees at both undergraduate and postgraduate levels.

The threshold entry points for professional qualification will have been set by a regulator such as the Health and Care Professions Council (HCPC) who regulate 16 health and social care professions in the UK (HCPC 2016a). The HCPC holds official registers for people who use legally protected titles including Dieticians, Clinical Scientists, Practitioner Psychologists and Radiographers. They approve pre-registration programmes in their domain and use their powers to protect the public by sanctioning and sometimes removing registrants who fall short of their standards through formal hearings as part of their Fitness to Practice Tribunal processes (see Chapter 1).

Pre-registration programmes are generally scrutinised against additional professional body standards or learning principles, such as those provided by the College of Paramedics (2014) or Royal College of Occupational Therapists (COT 2014). These bodies have an active interest in developing the knowledge base for their respective professions. They will offer to endorse programmes producing practitioners who can be regarded as fit for their profession. Some professions are approved by joint bodies who combine both regulatory and professional body functions such as the Nursing and Midwifery Council or the General Optical Council. This shows the quality that must be achieved by each new practitioner before they even start their first working day as a qualified professional.

In the UK, the growth and monitoring of knowledge and skill development as learning begins is very structured. For a student practitioner, rites of passage are through graded achievement in practice skills and academic work, typically marking the progress from year to year towards qualification. Whilst there may be some elements of choice for study within most pre-registration programmes (e.g. research project or elective placement), there is parity in achievement between institutions to gain a recognised exit award. To illustrate this, at the time of writing, in England, Northern Ireland and Wales a BSc (Hons) degree involves completion of 360 credits, equating to around 3600 hours of study over three years, whilst BSc (Hons) programmes in Scotland are structured over four years. Many students note this progress with pride, informally comparing their knowledge growth against that of newer students as they progress from year to year, or through formal reflections, whilst building up a CPD portfolio used to support their application for a first qualified practitioner post.

After they have qualified, CPD is an expectation of professional bodies and regulators embedded within Codes of Conduct and Ethics (e.g. HCPC 2016b; Nursing and Midwifery Council 2015; Society and College of Radiographers 2013; Chartered Society of Physiotherapy 2011). These bodies are clear that their members or registrants must engage in CPD activity to keep their knowledge and skills both up to date and relevant for their scope of practice, ensuring that they remain competent, confident and safe. They are also clear that this expectation does not stop regardless of the number of years someone has been qualified or the level of work undertaken throughout their career as a well-established or expert professional. This expectation is fair both to the people who use the services and to the employers who pay for the time of their staff. It is linked to the concept of professionalism and the level of integrity a professional person can offer. It reflects the nature of professional working, where knowledge and demands on practice change over time.

Whilst motivated and driven professionals may readily engage in plenty of ongoing CPD as a matter of course, and consider it part of their professional identity (Westcott 2005), all practitioners are required to meet minimum threshold standards in that regard. That said, CPD activity does not have to be carried out within a framework of credits or hours, like that needed to gain a formal academic qualification. Different health and social care professions have varying CPD requirements, which means that colleagues within an interprofessional team may each have different minimum thresholds for CPD.

The Nursing and Midwifery Council (NMC), for example, expects nurses and midwives to engage in a minimum of 35 hours' CPD every three years under their 'Revalidation' scheme. They expect a CPD log to be maintained to document this, and they require specified types of activity to be part of this mix, such as participatory CPD with other colleagues (not just self-managed study) (NMC 2016). On the other hand, HCPC registrants have no time recommendations to meet but, instead, may be randomly selected to have their personal CPD activity audited every two years. These types of mechanisms are designed to keep registrants mindful of the need to engage in CPD as required by the professional codes of ethics and conduct issued by these regulatory bodies (HCPC 2016b; NMC 2015).

Making time for vital updating and upskilling will help everyone on a professional register to demonstrate that their registration is a statement of their competence and currency. This is why it is so vital to retain the legally protected status of registered health or social care practitioner. Engaging in active CPD will help practitioners meet the clear expectations that service users have of any professionals – including contemporary expertise, informed reasoning and a high level of skill. Given that professional practitioners are registered personally (rather than under the name of their employer), and this is a public declaration of their competence, the importance of each practitioner maintaining their own CPD cannot be overstated. It is a professional duty for everyone to study, refresh and upskill every aspect of their practice.

Making the most of opportunities for CPD: Personal contributions, professional obligations and ensuring resilience

Some practitioners seem to make use of an abundance of CPD opportunities (sometimes known as Continuing Professional and Personal Development or CPPD) as part of their day-to-day professional practice, whilst others struggle to fit any of this into their busy working lives. It is interesting to consider what might influence this. Professional and regulatory body standards for students mean that all practitioners should graduate knowing the expectations for CPD placed upon them. They should also have learnt ways to recognise and reflect on new learning within their practice. In addition, they should be comfortable using and applying contemporary evidence to support their practice. Without these skills, arguably they would not achieve the standards of their baseline pre-registration programme at the point of graduation. It would therefore seem that everyone starts their working career meeting broadly similar expectations and with comparable skills in this area.

To help progress expectations for continued learning into practice, new practitioners should recognise when new learning is required to maintain or build upon their knowledge base at qualification. This enables practitioners to meet the demands of the scope of their practice as it moves on – an essential asset for a professional. They should know how to consult regularly with their own profession's literature or use supervision to reflect on developing skills, including those of professional or clinical reasoning. This is especially relevant as practitioners meet new or more complex situations, which is inevitable in this type of work.

Clearly, some working environments may be more conducive than others when allowing time for formal CPD within the working week, but this should not prevent anyone from advancing their CPD, whether within or outside working hours. Whilst some specific technical skills can only be learnt through practical experience in specialist work-based environments, few practitioners are isolated from peers and will usually be able to discuss developing their practice either face to face or online through professional social networking (see Chapter 7). There is generally easy access to quality evidence through professional body membership, relevant journals, thoughtfully selected sources on the internet and a range of further qualifications that can be accessed either through personal investment in CPD opportunities or with the support of an employer or other sponsor. Self-employed practitioners may even be able to offset the cost of their CPD activity against their UK tax return. Taking into account the difficulty of being released from employment for CPD, and the fact that more people are taking responsibility for their own development, many conferences and CPD courses are now available at weekends or online.

Some practitioners are looking at cost-effective ways to develop themselves and their colleagues, with activities that encourage critical examination of the most contemporary knowledge in their area of practice. Regular inhouse journal clubs, critical peer case reviews and master classes with invited experts within services can often be combined with working lunches or twilight/breakfast slots to accommodate busy service demands. Some practitioners engage in regular online debates with their peers, which can help people think through contemporary issues and network with other people in their specialty. Consistent activities of this type can help staff recognise and develop their knowledge and skill base, as well as working on gaps. Meeting with colleagues (with a specific agenda of mutual staff development) can work well in order to maintain confidence in topical trends for practice, even when services are intensely demanding on staff time.

Most staff are aware of formal staff development mechanisms used in bigger services like the NHS, such as professional supervision and annual appraisals or reviews for each employee. These are designed to help practitioners formally identify targets for CPD linked to the service need around them and can help engage the employer's support in meeting these needs. Some employers may offer newer practitioners a preceptorship scheme to help bridge the transition from student to registered professional. Where available, these can be well received and are recognised as being valuable in attracting, developing and retaining staff (Morley 2013).

Receiving less formal mentorship from a more experienced colleague may also support staff at all levels to develop themselves, away from the policy-driven supervision and appraisal protocols of their service. This mechanism is something that independent and more isolated practitioners can also arrange, as it provides a valuable opportunity to share some of the stresses and issues inherent in independent or more remote practice settings, thus enhancing career development. In this way, a more experienced colleague or practice expert can give guidance in areas of growth and professional progression, without being linked to the formally recorded performance objectives that often characterise supervision. Some professional bodies can also help practitioners to access a suitable mentor.

In addition to this more traditional model, 'modern mentoring' (Emelo 2015) is increasingly offering practitioners valuable support and opportunities for self-development. Mechanisms that include professionally orientated online engagement with peers, informal group meetings and other types of social media networking can help people exchange and share issues of mutual interest regarding skill development and professional growth. This is especially important for more isolated practitioners, but also offers much potential for everyone to widen their peer group, away from their workplace.

Such contacts with a peer group who share the same practice interest can be supportive and affirming and enhance resilience for practitioners who may be working in isolation, or do not have access to mentorship in their place of work. That said, care must be taken by all practitioners to remain within the scope of their given profession and the skill base appropriate to their job title and role when engaged in modern mentorship. Whilst employer-led schemes can be assumed to have considered this when offering mentorship arrangements at a local level, people engaged in modern mechanisms with online peers must take care to ensure this is maintained. Many allied health professions are aware that the scope of their profession and practice varies internationally, for example, and it is easy to assume that in the UK this is the same, but it is not always the case even with UK regulation processes. The four nations of the UK have different governance and policy structures that shape the practice and scope of local services, for instance (see Chapter 8). It is helpful to clarify whether online mentors have different contextual drivers and expectations in their workplace when discussing skills, knowledge and career development within the mentoring relationship. This can enhance knowledge of other localities and practice, whilst developing breadth of understanding and debate about professional issues.

Maintaining enthusiasm for your chosen profession and ensuring that you increase your confidence and skills will help you maintain a quality service for both your employer and your service users/patients. It is vital to maintain a positive view of your practice responsibilities and skills to ensure healthy engagement and longevity in your career. Many professional roles (including those in health and social care) can be stressful at times. Unexpected or unsupported levels of stress may mean that 'burnout' becomes a real risk. In this case, your view of your role may become a negative one and you may struggle to find the satisfaction and enjoyment that originally brought you into your profession (Clouston 2015).

Practitioners may feel overwhelmed by forces like change. They may struggle to devote time and energy to professional development. Practice may then be reduced to a functional level, lacking inspiration at best, with little motivation to improve or develop further. Importantly this loss of engagement and burnout can lead to poorer health and social care service provision. It could even mean condoning or falling into unacceptable practices that result in being reported to regulators like the NMC or HCPC.

To prevent this, we need to consider some wide-ranging questions:

- What makes some practitioners resilient and able to embrace change whilst others allow themselves to sink into the doldrums of negativity towards their profession, practice and employer?
- What enables some practitioners to work positively and well despite having negative peers around them?
- How can you maintain the 'good health' of your own professional practice and its values?

Being aware of (and ensuring) personal resilience is more vital than ever before and is linked to our ability to cope well with change. Many people are resilient when change is of their choosing, such as coping with the demands of a promotion, but then struggle to access or use these skills when change is imposed on them, such as a service redesign. We need to remember that health and social care systems are a huge budgetary commitment for the UK, and are therefore areas of key political interest for all governments, irrespective of political ideology. As such they have been subject to frequent change and restructuring for many years. With constant and ongoing drives for quality improvement alongside the need to save money, this seems set to continue. With all this in mind, resilience is clearly vital in order to work positively in this climate.

It is essential to have an understanding of how to gain and maintain resilience (see Chapter 15) and this can be achieved through a wide range of personal and professional actions or mechanisms. We all bring our own personality and skill set to professional practice, but we may not always understand how these can be used to accommodate and work with the opportunities that change brings. Without this understanding, we may fear the unknown, and this can lead to reactive, rather than proactive and considered practice, which may in turn be linked to negativity and poor work performance. Instead of waiting to see what is going to happen around us without any ownership of that process, we need to work to accommodate inevitable changes that will continue for many years. This will enhance our motivation.

Understanding the drivers of change, and the impact of changes, can really help practitioners make sense of reviews of practice and policy in large health and social care systems (see Chapters 6 and 8). It is therefore very helpful to find out as much as you can about what is going on and why decisions are being made. Regular engagement with quality news output and topical comment, such as professional body responses to key policy proposals, can help, as well as engaging in consultations and debate closer to home. Being an active member of your professional body, undertaking committee level duties within your organisation or working in an advisory capacity on local or wider projects can also help develop your understanding and generate ideas about how to work well in the context of change.

Working with colleagues to reflect and develop your practice to meet broader agendas can also help ensure that you feel you are embracing necessary change – for instance, developing use of more statistically valid and reliable outcome measures in a service where performance quality and work throughput are being questioned as part of an efficiency drive. Using supervision and mentorship that encourages your capacity for personal growth may help you discover just how and when you meet challenges with resilience, including evaluation of your expectations when working within a climate of change.

This should also involve examining your workload and the support you get, to ensure challenges are set at a level that is 'just right' in terms of your career development to date. This will encourage and enable your progression, rather than under-stimulate or overwhelm your efforts in the professional development sphere. It is also essential to ensure a varied work-life balance, to counterbalance experiences within your practice. Health and social care professionals often work with the most vulnerable, fragile and needy people in our society. Ensuring that you look after your own social and personal needs as part of a balanced lifestyle can make you a stronger and more resilient worker and help you thrive on the challenges and rewards that come from being a competent practitioner. Finally, in terms of your own resilience, it is important to be passionate and proud of your work; and securing an inspirational mentor or linking with colleagues who share your passion for practice can really help here.

It is also important to consider maintaining your resilience in terms of career progression. With this in mind, it is helpful to plan ahead when applying for promotions or accepting posts that demand more professional autonomy. More senior posts and independent practice inevitably mean that there is less support available when making important decisions, compared to working at an entry grade in a large well-staffed department. Many newly appointed senior practitioners may be surprised at the adjustments required within their own practice as their role alters and more junior staff look to them for guidance and support. As a manager or senior practitioner, you may need to make uncomfortable decisions that will not always be well received by your colleagues. You need to be able to respond and cope professionally when people question your decisions or your support for management directives, as well as helping others assimilate the impact of these within their workload.

Supervision is often more intermittent for senior staff and may not be profession specific in some areas as you move into specialist practice. Be prepared to look wider for mentoring or supervision. It may be helpful to consider seeking this help from different people for discrete areas of your senior practice such as management skills or highly technical skills. This is a useful area for discussion when applying for more senior posts if possible.

Conclusion

This chapter has explored the importance of becoming and remaining a responsible, autonomous practitioner. It has also highlighted the interest of a wide range of stakeholders (including regulators, professional, service providers and service users) in the quality of our ongoing professional growth. We have outlined how, after qualification, professional growth involves personal responsibility and embracing opportunities, many of which can be self-perpetuating. By outlining the importance of CPD and mechanisms such as mentoring, this chapter has shown how practitioners can maintain the momentum for growth that will help them throughout their career. The importance of resilience and the ability to work in a context of change have also been emphasised. This can all ensure that everyone who provides and uses health and social care services is afforded excellence and the best possible services.

Reflective questions

- Evaluate the characteristics, skills and experiences that you have noted in your colleagues that help them to be responsible and resilient practitioners.
    - How might you adopt or grow some of these qualities or skills?
    - How will you measure and monitor any success resulting from implementing these?
- Carefully reflect on the types of learning that work best for you. How can you better use these to keep your CPD updated in times of change when you have a heavy workload?

- If your regulator wanted evidence of your professional growth this week, are you confident you could deliver to their standards?
  - Analyse how you can make time for regular CPD activity (either within or outside working hours) that will ensure your development progresses and your skills remain up to date.
  - Consider what type of regular CPD activity you could do and how you will fit it into your schedule.

References

Chartered Society of Physiotherapy. (2011). *Code of Members' Professional Values and Behaviour.* London: Chartered Society of Physiotherapy. http://www.csp.org.uk/publications/code-members-professional-values-behaviour (last accessed 10.9.2016).

Clouston, T.J. (2015). *Challenging Stress, Burnout and Rust-out: Finding Balance in Busy Lives.* London: Jessica Kingsley.

College of Occupational Therapists. (2014). *Royal College of Occupational Therapists' learning and development standards for pre-registration education.* London: Royal College of Occupational Therapists.

College of Paramedics. (2015). *Paramedic Curriculum Guidance.* 3rd edn, revised. Bridgewater: College of Paramedics.

Emelo, R. (2015). *Modern Mentoring.* Virginia: ATD Press.

Health and Care Professions Council. (2016a). *About Us.* London: Health and Care Professions Council. http://hpc-uk.org/aboutus/ (last accessed 10.8.2016).

Health and Care Professions Council. (2016b). *Standards of conduct, performance and ethics Revised.* London: Health and Care Professions Council. http://hpc-uk.org/aboutregistration/standards/standardsofconductperformance andethics (last accessed 11.8.2016).

Morley, M. (2013). *Preceptorship Handbook for Occupational Therapists.* 3rd edn. London: College of Occupational Therapists.

Nursing and Midwifery Council (2015). *The Code: Professional standards of practice and behaviour for nurses and midwives.* London: Nursing and Midwifery Council. https://www.nmc.org.uk/globalassets/sitedocuments/nmc-publications/nmc-code.pdf (last accessed 11.8.2016).

Nursing and Midwifery Council. (2016). *Revalidation: How to revalidate with the NMC. Requirements for renewing your registration.* London: Nursing and Midwifery Council. https://www.nmc.org.uk/globalassets/sitedocuments/revalidation/how-to-revalidate-booklet.pdf (last accessed 15.9.2016).

Society and College of Radiographers. (2013). *Code of Professional Conduct.* London: The Society and College of Radiographers. http://www.sor.org/learning/document-library/code-professional-conduct (last accessed 9.4.2017).

Westcott, L. (2005). 'Continuing Professional Development' in *Working in Health and Social Care: An introduction for allied health professionals.* T.J. Clouston & L. Westcott (eds). Edinburgh: Elsevier Churchill Livingstone.

Section 2
Working together and communication

Introduction
By Steven W. Whitcombe

This section of the book addresses the importance of communication for effective health and social care practice. Communication itself is in a state of transition and the means by which we communicate with each other are continually evolving and subject to change.

Chapter 5 explores the concept of team working and the various types of team (such as multidisciplinary or uniprofessional) that you may be part of in your work environment. The structure and organisation of teams can differ in terms of size, complexity and function. However, the author of this chapter maintains that a professional and person-centred approach is an essential goal for any team in health and social care. The chapter considers the effectiveness of team working and the influence of human factors, such as 'personality traits', on team decision-making. It offers some practical tips for better team working and reflective questions that require you to think about the skills and knowledge that you bring to the teams with which you work.

Chapter 6 adopts a broader focus by exploring partnership working in health and social care. Historically, health and social care services were divided, with separate aims and purposes, but in response to current political pressure for more efficient and person-centred outcomes, these organisations (like others, such as housing and educational services) are now having to work together. This chapter takes a 'macro level' approach and considers the different forms of partnership working in the devolved nations of the United Kingdom. It also takes a 'meso level' approach by exploring types of local service agreements that require inter-agency working. The chapter discusses the challenges of partnership working, including the difficulties of combining models of care (i.e. medical or social models that reflect different professional values and philosophies). The chapter asks readers to think about issues of power when working in partnerships and to contemplate who benefits most from these arrangements.

Finally, Chapter 7 examines forms of communication in the digital age. As well as identifying who we communicate with, as health and social care professionals, it clarifies professional obligations in terms of appropriate communication, especially regarding relatively new forms of interaction such as social media. Moreover, the authors suggest that evolving mechanisms of communication (particularly digital) will continue to raise new questions about how to maintain professional boundaries when working with service users and their families. That said, the chapter also encourages you to reflect upon how you can embrace technology and new forms of communication to enhance service users' lives.

In order to get the most from these chapters, we ask that you really engage with and reflect on the questions and practical exercises you will find in them. It is only through an honest and meaningful exploration of your own beliefs and values that the full benefit of this reading will be experienced.

Chapter 5

Team working in complex organisations: Principles and practice

Tim Lewis

Learning outcomes

By the end of this chapter you will be able to:
- Reflect on the complexity of team working and discuss the differences between profession-specific and multiprofessional team working
- Discuss concepts such as delegation and supervision and identify how these are implemented in the workplace
- Recognise the influence of 'human factors and emotions' in the workplace and reflect on the challenges of remaining professional and effective when working in teams.

Introduction

If you are newly qualified, this chapter aims to help you adapt to your new role as a qualified, and professionally accountable, practitioner or therapist, and to understand the workings of your new team by exploring some fundamental questions relating to your practice. If you have been working for any length of time, this chapter will offer you an overview of the complexities of team working and help you to understand your role within the team.

Much of the research on team working was conducted during the latter half of the last century, when the fields of human resource management and the behavioural sciences were coming to the fore. It would be remiss, therefore, for this chapter to neglect the theoretical perspectives developed from some of these seminal works but, wherever possible, these perspectives will be augmented by more recent research findings and discussions of current policy initiatives.

There will, of necessity, be some crossover between themes discussed in this chapter and elsewhere in this book – for example, chapters discussing communication, professionalism and managing change. Where these overlaps occur, you will be cross-referred to the relevant chapters to enable you to explore these topics in greater depth.

What type of team are you joining?

This simple question can be broken down into several subsidiary considerations, all of which will have a bearing on your work within the team. For example: what is the purpose and scope of the team you are joining? Who makes up the team, and how large is it? Is it well established or newly formed, and what is its overriding culture?

Social researchers working in the 1990s differentiated between groups of people put together to form 'working groups' and true 'teams' (see Katzenbach & Smith 1993, for example). Using the criteria generated in this research, it follows that groups involving professionals working within health and social care can justifiably be classed as teams because of their individual, mutual and collective accountability, and because their work focuses on specific tasks (or cases) under the umbrella of the broader service delivery of the organisation. Furthermore, given that teams in health and social care are normally put together to provide a service for a client base over a period of time, they fit into the commonly accepted definition of an 'operational team' (Open University 2016). Within these teams, though, there may be a need for individuals to address a specific assignment in a given period of time – for example, dealing with an emergency referral. At times such as these, specialist expertise may be required, along with a degree of autonomous decision-making, to ensure the optimum outcome. In these circumstances, the team can demonstrate the attributes of a 'task culture', as described by Handy (1993).

Teams in health and social care can vary in size considerably, with some community-based teams consisting of a handful of professionals or, at the other extreme, departments in large teaching hospitals that consist of hundreds of professional and support staff. Each extreme has advantages and disadvantages, and the team's size will obviously affect the amount of time it takes to get to know and build the trusting relationships with colleagues that are essential to effective team working (Costa *et al.* 2001). Because it is easier to forge relationships in small groups, these teams are often more effective, as they encourage individuality and creativity (Choi 2013). The need for an all-encompassing *esprit de corps* may be less important, or achievable, in a larger team, which might affect the time it takes for a newcomer to develop their professional identity. Individuals have a need for social interaction so, in response to the risk of isolation in large teams, smaller subgroups will often develop. This is not always a positive development, as gaining membership of these subgroups, or cliques, can sometimes be problematic for the new team member.

Kelly and Barsade (2001) cite Bale's seminal (1950) observation that groups have both a functional and a social or emotional character, and it has been recognised for many years that acceptance into groups can depend not only on the skills that a person can contribute, but also their social 'attractiveness' (Blau 1960). Sweetman *et al.* (2013) have developed this concept of social integration further to demonstrate that the regard given to an individual within a group influences not only that person's status but can also affect the culture and motivation of that group.

However, social integration is less likely to cause problems in newly formed teams, as the relationships and status setting are still relatively fluid, as pointed out by Tuckman (1965). These factors become more firmly established in older teams and can be particularly difficult in teams that have been formed from previously separate teams – for example, when departments have been amalgamated. In these circumstances, differing team cultures often exist and it might be many years before complete integration of the teams occurs. Difficulties may also arise when different team members have varied or competing ambitions or aspirations, and this may provide an opportunity to develop your interpersonal (as well as your clinical or practice) skills.

Just as the health service has been reorganised in an attempt to reduce bureaucracy and improve flexibility and responsiveness in service delivery (Welsh Government 2013), so many organisations are recognising the advantages of small teams (Choi 2013). Anecdotal evidence suggests that the trend is to establish several smaller, task-focused teams within larger departments, thereby promoting an increased sense of responsibility and accountability in team members.

The composition of the team you are joining is also worth considering. The majority of teams within health and social care involve members of several disciplines working together (i.e. a multidisciplinary team) to provide a service for its client base. Although you may work in a department or service composed of members of just one professional discipline (for example, physiotherapy), the service users you are caring for are likely to be receiving care from members of a variety of disciplines. Each service user will work with both support workers as well as members of different professions, so you will still be working as part of a multidisciplinary team (MDT). For other professions, such as operating department practice (ODP), MDT working is a feature of everyday life as ODPs routinely practise alongside nurses, anaesthetists, surgeons, radiographers and so forth. Regardless of your chosen profession however, MDT working can present its own challenges.

The first of these is communication. In the past twenty years, a number of high-profile cases have raised serious concerns regarding governance and the interactions between different professions and agencies working in health and social care. These in turn have led to a huge emphasis on the importance of effective communication within and between teams (Kennedy 2001), especially in regard to the differing assumptions, jargon and priorities that are characteristics of different disciplines. This topic is discussed in greater depth in Chapter 6 of this book.

The communication issue is complicated further by the hierarchical nature and attendant power relationships of teams in health and social care. Professional groups have historically been organised in hierarchies, with the power largely focused on the holders of the most senior posts and the lowest levels being populated by students and the newly qualified (Walton 2006). Traditionally, communication within these hierarchies has followed the chain of command from the top downwards and, because the career progression of those on the lower levels is largely dependent on the goodwill of those on higher levels, those on lower levels can be reluctant to make their voices heard. This situation is slowly changing within health and social care as multidisciplinary working becomes more common, with initiatives such as *Five Steps to Safer Surgery* (National Patient Safety Agency 2009) encouraging improved multidisciplinary team working. That said, the structure of many larger health care organisations ensures that uniprofessional hierarchies continue to exert considerable influence.

Another challenge is the way in which the different professionals within the MDT work together. Among others, Hall and Weaver (2001) have suggested that the working of MDTs can be modelled along a continuum, dependent on the lines of communications, locus of decision-making and the collaboration between members of that team. Thylefors *et al.* (2005) used the terms 'multiprofessional', 'interprofessional' and 'transprofessional' to identify three models of MDT working along this continuum. The multiprofessional model is the most hierarchical, with a single point of command and very little communication occurring laterally between the team members. In interprofessional teams, professional boundaries are reasonably distinct, but communications and exchanges of ideas occur freely between team members. Finally, decision-making and professional role boundaries became blurred in the transprofessional model, where the individuals become better able to contribute to the work of each profession. In their study, Thylefors *et al.* (2005) surveyed Swedish operating theatre staff and found that the definition of MDTs in this area was quite fluid, with the majority of staff feeling that most of their work was conducted somewhere between interprofessional and transprofessional.

You may have had the opportunity to learn alongside students from different professions as part of your undergraduate education, and this might be a good opportunity to consider which model of multidisciplinary working was involved, and what impression that experience of MDT working left you with. In this author's experience, interprofessional education can initially take some students outside their comfort zones, especially when they are still developing confidence in their own professional identity. Most students respond more positively though, once they have experienced the realities of clinical professional practice. Barr and Low (2011) have suggested that effective interprofessional education typically:

- engenders interprofessional capability
- encourages the devising of outcome-led learning, delivering collaborative capabilities
- enhances practice within each profession
- enables each profession to improve its practice to complement that of others
- informs joint action to improve services and instigate change
- encourages the application of critical analysis to collaborative practice
- improves outcomes for individuals, families and communities
- enables practitioners to respond more fully to the needs of service users.

Reflective questions

- Thinking about what you have read so far, are you able to identify the different teams you have encountered in your working role/s thus far?
- If you work alongside different professional groups, how would you describe the composition and structure of these teams, e.g. multidisciplinary, uniprofessional or interprofessional?

What is your role within the team?

Before you can become a fully functional member of a team, it is important to consider your place within it. You may recall the team roles described by Belbin (Belbin Associates 2015). While these definitions may not equate precisely with the team you are working in, the classification does serve to remind us that all members of a team have their own unique strengths and weaknesses, and it is in your interest to be able to reflect on your own attributes as you develop within your new team.

It is also worth considering whether you have been brought in as an addition to the team, to work on a new project, or to replace another member of the team who has moved on. If you have been employed as an additional team member, it is likely that you will be met with open arms by members of an overworked, and possibly stressed team! There will be little time to bask in your newfound popularity though, as the downside of this situation is that you will probably be expected to become fully effective in a very short space of time, with little opportunity for mentoring or coaching by other team members. If you are replacing a popular or particularly effective team member, there is a risk that your performance or personality will be compared to theirs by other team members, so you will need to make an effort to establish your own identity as soon as possible. It is also good to be aware that your socialisation into the larger team might be delayed if you are focusing on a specific project, although this can be exciting and challenging as well as being an excellent addition to your curriculum vitae.

Tuckman used findings from his review of previous research into the working of teams to formulate a seminal four-stage model of team development: Forming, Storming, Norming and Performing (Tuckman 1965). You might have encountered this model previously, perhaps during your undergraduate education, but it is useful to reflect on these stages when considering your integration into a new work team. For example, your first few days will be taken up by finding out who's who in the team (*forming*). Having identified your colleagues and commenced your work role, you might occasionally experience some (hopefully minor) friction with other team members over your approach to your work or designated areas of responsibility (*storming*). Once these early teething troubles have been addressed, you should be able to identify common ground with the rest of the team, along with your role boundaries (*norming*), before settling into your new role and working (*performing*) productively alongside your colleagues.

Another concept that is intrinsically linked to team working is that of human factors, or non-technical skills. This concept has been written about by authors such as Flin (2000, 2007), originally in the context of workplace safety. However, human factors can be applied to many other aspects of team working, particularly the key areas of communications, teamwork, situational awareness, leadership and decision making that were identified in Flin's original work (Yule *et al.* 2008).

Flin (2000) asserts that a predictive and proactive approach should be taken to these factors to ensure safe practices. When root cause analysis (National Patient Safety Agency 2011) has been undertaken, following failures in health and social care, it is often found that it is organisational systems, or culture, rather than the specific acts or omissions of individuals that are to blame; see, for example, the Kennedy report (2001) into the deaths at the Bristol Royal Infirmary. Reason (2000), in his 'Swiss cheese' model of causation, supports the idea of organisational rather than individual culpability by suggesting that accidents frequently occur when a combination of relatively minor factors coincide, which then allow a far more significant error to occur.

In the light of these principles, a great deal of emphasis is now placed on the importance of individuals taking responsibility for their areas of work, being active participants in the decision-making process and voicing their concerns. Speaking out against practices that appear to be accepted as the norm by your colleagues can place you in a very uncomfortable position, especially if you are new and relatively junior within the department. However, you should remember that, according to the Health and Care Professions Council (HCPC 2016), reporting poor practice is a professional obligation, and failure to do so may not only endanger patients or clients, but also your registration. If your concerns are not acted upon, it may be necessary to escalate the matter by bringing it to the attention of senior managers or even an external authority; in these circumstances, you will be protected by law for 'whistleblowing' (Her Majesty's Government 2015). The preface of this book highlights one practitioner's story of voicing concerns linked to the crisis investigated by Francis (2013) at Mid Staffordshire Hospital.

Thankfully, the need to report poor practice is very rare. Generally speaking, teams within health and social care will have shared values and goals, and successes and achievements within the team will be celebrated by all. As in all human relationships, however, disagreements and interpersonal conflict can occasionally arise, and it is important for the efficient functioning of the team that these are managed promptly and effectively. Interpersonal conflict can take several forms; it can smoulder away for weeks or months, creating a general air of discomfort, or it can come out of nowhere like a flash of lightning. Some interpersonal conflict will simply be the result of a clash of personalities, in which case all you can do is to admit that you do not get along and try and work together as professionals. Other conflicts can be due to differences of opinion, or resentment over, for example, work allocations, or simple misunderstandings.

One frequent cause of ill feeling and conflict is the introduction of change. It is important to remember that change can be unsettling, especially for those who have established their practice and the way they manage their workload over a long period of time. If you are the person responsible for introducing a change in practice, it is essential to try and get existing staff to accept the necessity for change beforehand, as in the 'unfreezing' phase of Lewin's (1958) change model (cited in Levasseur 2001).

However it manifests itself, interpersonal conflict will always have an emotional component, and it is crucial to recognise the presence of this in both parties, and separate it from more objective issues. Underman-Boggs (2015) asserts that if conflict is managed well (for instance, with honesty and maturity), it can be used to aid team development. The following key stages in conflict resolution are outlined (Underman-Boggs 2015):

1. Identify conflict issues
2. Know your own response to conflict
3. Separate the problem from the people involved
4. Stay focused on the issue
5. Identify available options
6. Try to identify established standards to guide the decision-making process.

As part of your role, even if you are newly qualified, you may well be required to supervise the work of other staff, such as junior members of your own profession, students or support staff. Just as you are accountable to your regulatory body for your own actions, you must remember that when you delegate a task to another, you are still accountable for that person's performance of that task (HCPC 2016; Nursing & Midwifery Council 2015). For this reason, when delegating a task to a person, you must also ensure that the person is suitably trained and authorised by their employer to undertake that task. Many support staff, in particular, are confident and appear to be very competent, so it can be easy to forget the defined limitations of their roles. This is a potential pitfall of the transprofessional model of working discussed earlier.

Reflective questions

- What aspects of your new role or existing role (if any) could you delegate to others?
- How ready are you to supervise the work of others?
- Is there an opportunity for you in your current role to develop the skills needed for effective supervision?

What support is available to you in your new role?

You have survived your first week in your new post; the caseload is challenging but enjoyable, and your colleagues are friendly and seem to be very capable. What else do you need to know?

You should have been informed of who your line manager is, and hopefully they will have arranged some form of induction programme for you in your first few days. It is a good idea to meet up with your line manager soon after you commence in post in order to help with your orientation, to set ground rules about expected behaviour, health and safety and other key policies, and to give you the opportunity to ask any questions you had meant to ask before, but hadn't quite got round to. You may well be subject to a probationary period, so it is most important that you find out what this involves, especially in relation to any assessment that may be required before your post can be considered substantive. You should also aim to find out about appraisal schemes, annual leave entitlement and sickness monitoring procedures (ACAS 2015). Most employers in health and social care adhere to good employment practices, but you might find it helpful to gain additional information from your professional body or trade union in this regard.

Many employers, especially in the NHS, will also run a preceptorship scheme, under which new staff will be allocated to a more experienced staff member who can guide them through their first few months in their new role (Department of Health 2009). While work pressures may make it difficult for this scheme to be followed in every detail, having an experienced member of staff to coach you in the finer points of departmental policy and practice is invaluable.

The extent to which schemes such as preceptorship are adhered to can also depend on the culture of the department in which you work, and this is an area in which you, as a newly qualified practitioner, can be proactive. As registered professionals, you and your colleagues are required to engage in continuing professional development (CPD) in order to ensure that your 'skills and knowledge [are] up to date' and you are 'able to work safely, legally and effectively' (HCPC 2012, p.1). Humphris and Masterson (2000) suggest that CPD should be part of an individual's life-long learning and that, in order for this to be encouraged in professional practice, workplaces should aim to develop a learning culture. They continue to suggest that learning cultures promote reflection and adaptability among their staff (Humphris & Masterson 2000), which in turn may lead to patient/client benefits through the introduction of small-scale quality improvements, as recommended by the 1000 Lives Plus organisation (1000 Lives Plus 2012).

Conclusion

It has probably been said many times before that the transition from being a student undertaking supervised practice to being a qualified and professionally accountable practitioner and working as part of a care team can sometimes feel quite daunting.

Productive team working is influenced by many factors, including organisational culture, interpersonal relationships, effective communication and sharing of common goals, which in health and social care must be focused on the service user or patient. When teams are composed of more than one professional discipline, responsibility and decision-making will often be shared but care needs to be taken to ensure that members work within professional boundaries and their individual scope of practice, especially when tasks are delegated. While we may occasionally encounter difficulties working with individual team members, it is our professional responsibility to ensure that any differences are resolved and our service users/patients receive the highest quality care or therapy at all times.

Reflective questions

- What qualities and skills do you bring to the team working?
- How do you measure the effectiveness of the teams in which you work?

References

1000 Lives Plus. (2012). *The 1000 lives plus quality improvement guide for educators and students*. Cardiff. 1000 Lives Plus.

ACAS (2015). *Starting staff: induction*. http://www.acas.org.uk/media/pdf/3/0/Starting-staff-induction.pdf (last accessed 25.4.2016).

Barr, H. & Low, H. (2011). *Principles of Interprofessional Education*. https://www.caipe.org/resources/publications/barr-low-2011-principles-interprofessional-education/ (last accessed 11.8.2016).

Belbin Associates (2015). *Belbin team roles*. http://www.belbin.com/about/belbin-team-roles/ (last accessed 11.8.2016).

Blau, P.M. (1960). A Theory of Social Integration. *American Journal of Sociology*. **65** (6), 545–56.

Choi, J. (2013). *The Science Behind Why Small Teams Work More Productively: Jeff Bezos' 2 Pizza Rule*. https://blog.bufferapp.com/small-teams-why-startups-often-win-against-google-and-facebook-the-science-behind-why-smaller-teams-get-more-done (last accessed 11.8.2016).

Costa, A.C., Roe, R.A. & Taillieu, T. (2001). Trust within teams: The relation with performance effectiveness. *European Journal of Work and Organisational Psychology*. **10** (3), 225–44.

Department of Health (2009). *Preceptorship Framework for Newly Registered Nurses, Midwives and Allied Health Professionals*. London: Department of Health.

Flin, R., Mearns, K., O'Connor, P. & Bryden, R. (2000). Measuring safety climate: identifying the common features. *Safety Science*. **34** (1–3), 177–92.

Flin, R. (2007) Measuring safety culture in healthcare: A case for accurate diagnosis. *Safety Science*. **45**, 653–67.

Francis, R. (2013). *Report of the Mid Staffordshire NHS Foundation Trust Public Inquiry* http://www.midstaffspublicinquiry.com/ (last accessed 5.6.2016).

Hall, P. & Weaver, L. (2001). Interdisciplinary education and teamwork: a long and winding road. *Medical Education*. **35** (9), 867–75.

Handy, C. (1993). *Understanding organizations*. 4th edn. London: Penguin Books Ltd.

Health and Care Professions Council (2012). *Your guide to our standards for continuing professional development*. London: Health and Care Professions Council.

Health and Care Professions Council (2016). *Standards of conduct, performance and ethics*. London: Health and Care Professions Council.

Her Majesty's Government (2015). *Whistleblowing for employees*. https://www.gov.uk/whistleblowing/who-to-tell-what-to-expect (last accessed 25.04.2016).

Humphris, D. & Masterson, A. (2000). *Developing new clinical roles: a guide for health professionals*. Edinburgh: Churchill Livingstone.

Katzenbach, J.R. & Smith, D.K. (March/April 1993). The discipline of teams. *Harvard Business Review*. 111–20.

Kelly, J. & Barsade, S. (2001). Mood and Emotions in Small Groups and Work Teams. *Organizational Behavior and Human Decision Processes*. **86** (1), 99–130.

Kennedy, I. (2001). *The report of the public inquiry into children's heart surgery at the Bristol Royal Infirmary 1984-1995: learning from Bristol*. http://webarchive.nationalarchives.gov.uk/+/www.dh.gov.uk/en/Publicationsandstatistics/Publications/PublicationsPolicyAndGuidance/DH_4005620 (last accessed 11.8.2016).

Levasseur, R.E. (2001). People skills: change management tools — Lewin's change model. *Interfaces*. **31** (4), 71–73.

National Patient Safety Agency (2009). *Five Steps to Safer Surgery*. http://www.nrls.npsa.nhs.uk/EasySiteWeb/getresource.axd?AssetID=93286 (last accessed 11.08.2016).

National Patient Safety Agency (2011). *Root Cause Analysis Investigation Training Materials*. http://www.nrls.npsa.nhs.uk/resources/collections/root-cause-analysis/rca-training-course-overview/ (last accessed 11.08.2016).

Nursing and Midwifery Council. (2015). *The Code: Professional standards of practice and behaviour for nurses and midwives.* London: Nursing and Midwifery Council.

Open University (2016). *How teams work. 1.2: operational teams.* http://www.open.edu/openlearn/money-management/management/leadership-and-management/how-teams-work/content-section-1.2 (last accessed 11.8.2016).

Reason, J. (2000). Human error: models and management. *British Medical Journal*. **320** (7237), 768–770.

Sweetman, J., Spears, R., Livingstone, A.G. & Manstead, A.S.R. (2013). 'Admiration regulates social hierarchy: Antecedents, dispositions, and effects on intergroup behavior'. *Journal of Experimental Social Psychology*. **49** (3), 534–42.

Thylefors, I., Persson, D. & Hellström D. (2005). Team types, perceived efficiency and team climate in Swedish cross-professional teamwork. *Journal of Interprofessional Care*. **19** (2), 102–14.

Tuckman, B.W. (1965). Developmental sequence in small groups. *Psychological Bulletin*. **63** (6), 384–99.

Underman-Boggs, K. (2015). 'Resolving Conflicts between Nurse and Client' in E.C. Arnold & K. Underman-Boggs (eds). *Interpersonal Relationships: Professional Communications Skills for Nurses*. 7th edn. St Louis: Elsevier.

Walton, M.M. (2006). Hierarchies: the Berlin Wall of patient safety. *Quality and Safety in Health Care*. **15**, 229–230.

Welsh Government (2013). *Transforming Health Improvement in Wales: Working together to build a healthier, happier future.* Cardiff: Welsh Government.

Yule, S., Rowley, D., Flin, R., Maran, N., Youngson, G., Duncan, J. & Paterson-Brown, S. (2009). Experience matters: comparing novice and expert ratings of non-technical skills using the NOTSS system. *Australian and New Zealand Journal of Surgery*. **79**, 154–60.

Chapter 6

Partnership working

Alison Strode

Learning outcomes

By the end of this chapter you will be able to:
- Explain why partnership working is central to public policy
- Examine the role of power in partnership working
- Discuss who benefits from partnership working
- Reflect on some different perspectives on partnership working.

Although partnership working is applicable to all areas of welfare, this chapter will focus on its application in health and social care. In recent years, there has been recognition that the NHS and social care services need to work in a much more coordinated way, not just with each other but also with other sectors such as education and housing. Repeated commitments to bring down the 'Berlin Wall' between health services and social care have led to partnership working increasingly being seen as a central feature of public services (Hansard 1997). The historical division of responsibilities between health and social care rests on distinguishing between:

- those who have 'health needs' and consequently receive a service that is free at the point of delivery
- those who are frail or disabled and have a 'social care' need, and consequently attract a means-tested local authority charge.

However, this distinction is highly contentious: partnership working has therefore been hailed as a way of creating more seamless boundaries between the two sectors.

Partnership working is seen as:

- providing more coherent and effective service delivery

- being more responsive to service users' needs
- adding value through agencies working together
- creating a shared culture
- enhancing the understanding of different professional roles.

Partnership working is not a new concept but continuing problems of organisational fragmentation and lack of continuity of services for those with health and social care needs have raised concerns about whether it is producing the benefits that it is supposed to deliver.

These concerns include:

- structural fragmentation (between and within health and social care services)
- procedural (differences in planning rounds)
- financial (differences in funding and resource mechanisms)
- professional (the difficulty of combining medical and social models)
- practical implications of working across organisational and professional boundaries.

(Adapted from Brechin *et al.* 2000, p.254)

Reflective questions

- Reflecting on your place of work, consider what forms of partnership working does your organisation engage with?
- What benefits (if any) does partnership working have for you?

What is partnership working?

There seems to be no general agreement about the definition of the term 'partnership working'. For instance, it would appear that there is a wide assortment of terms, including 'collaboration', 'multi-agency working', 'integration', 'networking' and 'joint working', which generally describe partnership working and which advocate cross-organisational and cross-agency working (Cook 2015).

The difficulties of defining the term 'partnership' are partly due to the fact that it seems to mean different things to different people. Dickinson and Glasby (2010, p.815) identified partnership working as:

> negotiation between people from different agencies committed to working together over more than the short term, [which] aims to secure the delivery of benefits or added value which could not have been provided by any single agency acting alone or through the employment of others and includes a formal articulation of purpose and plan to bind partners together.

The simplest of these definitions was cited by Lester *et al.* (2008, p.494) as 'any situation in which people work across organisational boundaries towards some positive end'.

Based on these definitions, it is clear that partnership working in every context has some common characteristics that will lead to desirable goals, including good use of resources and positive outcomes for service users.

Why is it central to public policy?

The Conservative governments of the 1980s and early 1990s created what were viewed as fragmented single agencies, driven by market-driven incentives that required better performance, especially in relation to costs and service users' needs. Consequently, this sort of approach was seen to aggravate the difficulties of dealing with complex problems, as the incentives to achieve organisational aims were greater than those of a more multi-agency approach. The arrival of a new Labour government in 1997 brought with it the intention to move from a contract culture to one based on partnership. Legislation, such as the Health Act (1999), sought to sweep away legal obstacles to partnership working by allowing the nomination of a partner to lead commissioning, pooled budgets and integrated provision of care. It brought with it financial incentives from central government funds that could only be accessed through multi-agency bidding.

The policy-making process has changed significantly over the last couple of decades, with central government no longer being the dominant player in the policy arena. The boundaries between the public and the private sphere have become blurred and a model of governance is emerging in which the government is just one participant among many involved in policy-making. More local and collaborative forms of organisation are also involved (Dickinson & Glasby 2010). The impact that this has had on health and social care has been to encourage not just collaboration between services such as education and youth justice in children's services but also between professionals and users of the various services (Glasby & Dickinson 2014).

Policy and legislation on partnership working

Since the late 1990s, devolution has led to the development of different structures for delivering partnership working in the different countries making up the UK and, consequently, different legislation.

England

NHS bodies and local authorities in England can pool budgets, combine their staff and management structures or delegate commissioning responsibilities to each other through section 75 of the NHS Act (2006). Section 75 of the NHS Act (2006) and, more recently, the Health and Social Care Bill (2012) established health and well-being boards in every local authority area to co-ordinate the commissioning of health and social care and promote greater scope for the integration of services across health and social care. However, some of the complexity of implementing the Bill came from the fragmenting of commissioning responsibility to around 400 separate local organisations such as Clinical Commissioning Groups, NHS England and Local Authorities (Humphries & Wenzel 2015).

Scotland

Within Scotland, the partnership agenda has become more prominent, with a clear shift towards mandatory partnerships. The Community Care and Health (Scotland) Act (2002) introduced key new provisions on joint working, which required each local authority and health board to set up a local partnership agreement that enabled partnerships to make payments to one another, to delegate functions to one another and, furthermore, to pool their budgets. Further legislation (the NHS Reform (Scotland) Act 2004) required NHS Boards to set up community health partnerships to co-ordinate the planning and provision of local health services, including mental health. More recent legislation, namely the Public Bodies (Joint Working) (Scotland) Act 2014 (Scottish Government 2015), has required health boards and local authorities to integrate health and social care services either by delegating to an Integration Joint Board or by the health board or local authority taking the lead responsibility for planning and resourcing service provision for adult health and social care services.

Wales

In Wales, health boards and local authorities are able to pool budgets, integrate teams and jointly commission services through Section 33 of the National Health Services (Wales) Act (2006). The ten-year plan for social care, *Sustainable Social Services*, published in 2011, also included plans to drive integration, for instance by requiring councils and health boards to jointly commission and arrange reablement services, to support people to regain independence. Part 9 of the Social Services and Well-being Act (2014) includes a duty to promote co-operation with partners to drive service delivery. Local authorities and health boards must work together to assess the care and support needs (and carer support needs) of the population in their area (Welsh Government 2015).

Northern Ireland

In contrast to the other UK countries, in Northern Ireland health and social care services are structurally integrated. All health and social care is commissioned by the Department of Health (Northern Ireland), and most services are delivered by five integrated health and social care trusts. The most recent legislation appertaining to partnership working is the Health and Social Care (Reform) Act (Northern Ireland) (2009). The rationale behind the reform of the health and social care system is to put in place structures which are patient-led, patient-centred and responsive to the needs of patients, clients and carers as well as being more effective and efficient. Partnership working is viewed as vital in order to reduce health inequalities and develop more productive working between public health, health and social care and local government. This is borne out in the strategic framework for public health, *Making Life Better: A Whole System Framework for Public Health 2013–2023*' (DHSSPS (NI) 2014) and the Bengoa Report, *Systems not Structure: Changing Health and Social Care* (2016) as well as *Health and Well-being 2026: Delivering Together* (Department of Health (NI) 2017).

What are the benefits of partnership working?

Partnerships are designed to support, encourage or enforce collaborative working within and between statutory and other sectors. Partnership working is seen as having the potential to improve value for money by removing overlap in the delivery of services (Balloch & Taylor 2001). It also helps to drive out waste and inefficiency and enables organisations to harness their collective purchasing power (collaborative advantage) to make effective use of economies of scale (Huxham & Vangen 2005). For health and social care, this results in making better use of public money and ensuring better outcomes for service users.

In 2005, the English Audit commission suggested that partnership working could help to deliver co-ordinated services to individuals to tackle complex or 'wicked' issues (Hudson 2010). Wicked issues arise when there is no simple approach to solving a problem because of multiple, sometimes competing, perspectives and because the problem may have several possible solutions. An example of this can be observed in care of older adults which requires collaboration amongst local agencies such as health, social care and the voluntary sector (Ferlie *et al.* 2013). Partnership working can reduce the impact of organisational fragmentation, allow access to new resources and help make better use of current resources. It can also align services with the needs of users, improving quality and stimulating more creative approaches to problems, as well as influencing the behaviour of the partners to achieve what could not be done if acting alone (Glasby *et al.* 2011).

However, there are several principles that are pertinent if partnerships are to be successful. These include and are dependent upon:

- the degree to which there is either a history of partnership working or the recognition that there is a need to work in partnership
- the level of engagement and visible commitment of the partners
- agreement about shared vision, values, aims and objectives

- high levels of trust, reciprocity and respect
- favourable environmental factors, such as financial support and a lack of cumbersome bureaucracy
- accountability
- adequate leadership and management.

(Adapted from Dowling et al. 2004)

The most important of these principles is viewed as being the development and maintenance of trust and the evidence shows that partnerships will work well where there is equivalent status (Asthana *et al.* 2002). Partnerships that have developed organically, because the partners themselves identified the need for the partnership, have been found to be more robust and meaningful than those formed in response to policy directives (Hunter & Perkins 2014). For example, in the context of health and social care, there is a long history of partnership working for services such as mental health, learning disabilities, older people and children through the establishment of joint consultative committees made up of members of local authorities and the health sector and the subsequent evolution into joint care planning teams (Baggott 2013).

Policymakers take it for granted that partnership working will reduce wasteful duplications and make more effective use of resources allocated to different agencies. Inter-agency and interprofessional collaboration will result in a more comprehensive response to the needs of individual patients or groups of clients, both at the planning stage and during delivery of services. So, is this the reality of partnership working?

Barriers to partnership working

A number of factors have been identified as creating barriers to successful partnership working. These are listed below.

Organisational factors:

- Competing organisational visions and differences in resource and spending criteria between local authorities and NHS partners are thought to undermine the aims of partnership working (Cameron & Lart 2014).
- Staff being located on separate sites can impede communication and sharing of information (Cameron *et al.* 2012).
- Not being clear about desired outcomes, and inaccurately calling things 'partnerships' to make them more acceptable, such as market-based public/private initiatives (Dickinson & Glasby 2010).

Cultural and professional factors:
- cultural clashes between people who come from different sorts of organisations, which can lead to inflexibility (Wildridge *et al.* 2004)
- lack of trust and respect (Glendinning *et al.* 2002)
- introductions such as the single assessment process, which require confidence in the assessments being made by others (Cameron & Lart 2014)
- partners being perceived as having an unequal status, such as imbalances of power in the hospital sector (Glasby & Dickinson 2014)
- competition for power in interprofessional working, sometimes due to lack of clarity about roles (Hudson 2002).

Government factors:
- compulsory government initiatives such as forced partnerships, where there is an insistence on agencies working together when the internal dynamic for collaboration might be weak (Hudson 2010)
- the use of targets, incentives and ring-fenced funding are ways for central government to steer and direct the actions of care agencies rather than ways of enabling them to co-operate to meet local needs (Glendinning *et al.* 2002).

All these potential barriers mean that, in practice, partnership working can sometimes be frustrating and tricky. This is because partnerships may operate at different levels and partners may have different motivations for engaging in them.

Whose interests are being served in partnership working?

Before answering this question about whose interests are being served, it is important to gain an understanding of the way power and authority is asserted and negotiated in partnerships in order to appreciate how different partners participate in and influence decision-making. Understanding what affects the delivery of health and social care involves recognising and acknowledging the existence of powerful groupings which have their own interests to pursue. Some examples of powerful groupings in health and social care include individual professions, professional associations, trade unions, local authorities, and regulators or managers in health service organisations – both public and private.

A good starting point for understanding power relations in partnership working is to read *Power – a radical view* (Lukes 2005). According to Lukes, power influences who gets what and when, and how one person can coerce another in a manner that is contrary to that person's interest. This coercion can be applied covertly or overtly. In his view, there are three dimensions to power, as listed below.

First dimension

The first dimension involves power shifts of uneven direct confrontations between parties where power and control are explicitly and openly displayed. It involves decision-making: for example, the ability to coerce another person to do something they would not otherwise do. In issues of conflict, whichever actor can claim to have the prevailing culture on their side can further strengthen their position.

Second dimension

The second dimension involves an indirect contest of power between parties. Lukes (2005) calls this the 'mobilisation of bias' where, by commanding, controlling, setting and influencing the rules of the situation, as well as dissuading actions and agenda-setting, coercion, influence or manipulation, a situation of non-decision-making arises in which conflict can be suppressed before it is even voiced. It is evident in the 'mobilisation of bias' that a set of predominant values, beliefs, rituals and institutional procedures (which may be called 'rules of the game') operate systematically and consistently – to the benefit of certain individuals and groups and at the expense of others.

Third dimension

The third dimension encompasses control and influence over what the less powerful party thinks and what they understand of the world and of their own interests. Lukes (2005) calls this 'latent conflict'. It involves the values and preferences of the less powerful being shaped by those exercising power, with those excluded possibly not even being conscious of where their own interests lie.

To encourage successful partnership working, the power dynamics of the partnerships and the fundamental inequalities between the partners need to be understood. Partnerships have been identified at three levels:

- macro level, which take place within a national or state ministry or at a country level
- meso level, which take place on a local service professional level
- micro level, which relate to individual service users' needs.

Government interests/the role of governance

At a macro level, partnership working theoretically signifies a departure from central government steering in favour of governance, which involves the reconfiguration of relationships between the state, civil society, the public and private sectors, citizens and communities and a diffusion of power away from the state. The view of Cook (2015, p.4) is that the 'focus on governance has been a direct response to the failure of 'command and control' and market approaches' in addressing complex social issues. Central to this way of working is the devolution of power and decision-making to local communities and for local government to shift from controlling to more co-ordinating and enabling approaches. Consecutive governments have assumed that partnership working can make a significant contribution to communities arriving at shared goals.

However, it has been identified in Lukes' (2005) second dimension of power that powerful partners can influence agendas through partnership working. For instance, the over-prescriptive encouragement of partnership working from central government has in some ways enabled policy-makers to avoid crucial issues involving irreconcilable structures and limited resources by giving practitioners the responsibility of mitigating the effects (Loxely 1997). Furthermore, partnership working can be seen as an effective means of ensuring that the state retains and, in some cases, strengthens its powers. These powers include dictating that organisations work in partnership, controlling what is up for consideration and also controlling what is resourced. This has the effect of reinforcing the power inequalities that already exist (Glendinning *et al.* 2002). In health and social care, for example, this can result in issues that are important to central government (such as targets for reducing teenage pregnancies) being given more priority in areas where this is actually less of a problem. The focus thus becomes meeting government targets rather than resolving local issues (Hunter & Perkins 2014).

The government can also be viewed as utilising Lukes' (2005) third dimension of power, whereby it has the power to shape people's desires and aspirations and define the terms within which public debates take place. Balloch and Taylor (2001) observe that partnership working has largely left existing power relations intact, thus enabling government partners to determine the rules of the game.

Professionals' interests

At a meso level, professionals are viewed as being committed to the provision of expert services and advice and their expert knowledge gives them power and authority. They are seen as more creative, altruistic and driven by ethical commitment as well as having a distinct identity due to being members of a profession (Clouston & Whitcombe 2008, Greenwood 1957). A profession that has attained a large measure of autonomy will seek to influence the policy of the state. In health care, the medical profession has a particularly powerful presence, influencing government policy through professional association representation on government committee inquiries and parliamentary debates. However, research suggests that the boundaries between professions have shifted and become more flexible in response to strategic, structural and organisational changes (Willis 2006). The tactics used by professions to protect or maintain their boundaries may involve both compromise and competition with rival professions (Abbott 1998). This can provide opportunities for other health care professions, such as allied health professionals or nurses, to renegotiate their power base by expanding their clinical roles and responsibilities.

Reflective questions

- Is it important to retain your professional identity when working with others?
- If so, how do you do this in response to increased levels of integrated working?
- To what extent are you able to utilise power to successfully compete with others for scarce resources?

Governments have been suggesting for some time that there should be more flexibility in the workforce and less working in professional silos (Department of Health 2000, Hall 2005). The prevailing political environment means that the power of professionals is viewed as being under threat. In this context, it can be seen that partnership working raises a number of difficulties for professionals which need to be considered, such as the loss of autonomy. The health professions will argue that their practitioners can be trusted to put the interests of clients or patients before their own and this is defended against the state in the setting of professional standards. However, all professions will compete and struggle for control over their work processes (Abbott 1998).

Lukes' (2005) second dimension of power can be seen in the power being exerted by the professional in taking control of the agenda of service users. This may be achieved by making certain issues taboo, manipulating the norms, rules and procedures that regulate agenda-setting, or forbidding certain participants to enter the decision-making arena altogether. Examples of this might include protecting general dominance through the use of professional language, both by staff and in official documentation (Furber & Thomson 2010). Alternatively, it might manifest in less powerful participants deciding not to 'make an issue' of something, as they calculate that they will be defeated. This has the effect of making the relationships unequal and therefore contributes to the failure of partnerships.

The state provides the funds and, to a degree, defines the activities of the caring professions. However, from the outset, there has been confusion about boundaries between the NHS and local authorities. In practice, power in the NHS and local authorities is so entrenched (Malin 2000) that it can be seen that Lukes' second dimension of power can be exercised by these powerful partners. This has allowed scope for denying responsibility, and consequently contributed to the 'silo' mentality, which enables professionals to simply 'pass the buck' across health and social care boundaries.

Using the care of older adults as an example, this can be contextualised for each of the four countries in the UK. For instance, health is largely free at the point of delivery in all four countries, whereas social care is delivered through market-led purchasing organisations (local authorities), delivered by private provider organisations. This can lead to arguments over whether service users have a health need (free care) or a social care need (paid care). Each country has its own approach to who pays what, based on assessment of need. In England, for example, local authorities will have their own charging policies, based on a financial assessment of what is reasonably practicable for an individual to pay. Meanwhile, in Scotland, personal care (such as washing and shaving) is free but in Wales people may be asked to pay for these services – up to a maximum cost of £60 per week.

Users' and carers' interests

The ultimate goal of partnership working should be for citizens, service users and communities to be active participants in services, rather than passive recipients who have been marginalised from exercising power.

When partnerships work well for service users, they can provide a more holistic approach to choosing services that best suit their needs. Features of partnership working that make a difference to services users and carers are:

- co-location of services, which enhances the responsiveness of the service
- multidisciplinary teams, so that both health and social care needs can be met
- extended partnerships that extend into other sectors, such as housing and the voluntary sector.

(Adapted from Petch *et al.* 2013)

While some claim that partnership working is a helpful way of responding to the needs of service users, others see it as leading to a concentration of power in the hands of service providers (Glasby & Dickinson 2014). Service users may be able to wield first-dimension power, in terms of expressing preferences or giving feedback. However, they are less able to wield power at the second dimension, regarding choice about the types of care that may be offered. In the third dimension, service users might not realise that they even have a role to play in decision-making regarding services, and are therefore likely to leave it to the professionals involved (Brechin *et al.* 2000).

Evidence has shown that if service users were able to truly exercise power over service developments, their priorities would be different from those of the relevant professions and organisations (Rummery 2009). Different user involvement methods are required to secure active user participation in decision-making at individual, care group and organisational levels (Tritter & McCallum 2006); and service users have a particular role to play in the framing of problems and not just designing solutions.

Thus it can be seen that all three of Lukes' (2005) dimensions of power are at play and can be used to illuminate the shifting patterns of dominance, alliance and conflict, as the various partners struggle to establish and maintain autonomy and control of their challenging and ever-changing environment.

Conclusion

There are some signs of progress, in that people are no longer questioning whether partnership working is the way forward. However, establishing and getting the best out of sustainable partnership working is more of a challenge. This chapter has set out to provide an overview of some of the key issues, including identifying the benefits of and barriers to partnership working and how power may be used by various stakeholders. It has also highlighted the fact that partnership working takes place at a number of levels, from local to national, and therefore the management of the diverse environment in which we live requires that the professions and agencies involved in health and social care all work together so that partnerships can be used for the greater good.

Reflective questions

- Think about all the different organisations and agencies that you work with. Who benefits from these arrangements and in what ways?
- How can we involve more service users in decision-making processes involving the services they utilise?

References

Abbott, A. (1988). *The system of professions. An essay on the division of expert labour.* Chicago: University of Chicago Press.

Asthana, S., Richardson, S. & Halliday, J. (2002). Partnership working in public policy provision: a framework for evaluation. *Social Policy and Administration.* **36** (7), 780–95.

Baggott, R. (2013). *Partnerships for public health and well-being.* Hampshire: Palgrave Macmillan.

Balloch, S. & Taylor, M. (2001). *Partnership working, policy and practice.* Bristol: Policy Press.

Bengoa, R., Stout, A., Scott, B., McAlinden, M. & Taylor M.A. (2016). Systems, *Not Structures: Changing Health and Social Care. Expert Panel Report.* https://www.health-ni.gov.uk/sites/default/files/publications/health/expert-panel-full-report.pdf (last accessed 5.7.2017).

Brechin, A., Brown, H. & Eby, M. (2000). *Critical practice in health and social care.* London: Sage.

Cameron, A., Lart, R., Bostock, L. & Coomber, C. (2012). Factors that promote and hinder joint and integrated working between health and social services. Social Care Institute for Excellence, *Research Briefing.* **41**, 1–23.

Cameron, A. & Lart, R. (2014). Service user and carers' perspectives of joint and integrated working between health and social care. *Journal of Integrated Care.* **22** (2), 62–70.

Clouston, T.J. & Whitcombe, S.W. (2008). The professionalisation of occupational therapy: a continuing challenge. *British Journal of Occupational Therapy.* **71** (8), 314–20.

Cook, A. (2015). *Partnership working across UK public services*. Edinburgh: What Works Scotland.

Department of Health (Northern Ireland) (2017). *Health and Well-being 2026 Delivering Together.* https://www.health-ni.gov.uk/sites/default/files/publications/health/health-and-well-being-2026-delivering-together.pdf (last accessed 5.7.2017).

Department of Health (1999). *Health Act.* London: The Stationery Office.

Department of Health. (2000). *The NHS Plan.* London: The Stationery Office.

DHSSPSNI (2014). *Making life better – a whole system strategic framework for public health 2013–2023*. https://www.health-ni.gov.uk/articles/making-life-better-strategic-framework-public-health (last accessed 30.9.2017).

Dickinson, H. & Glasby, J. (2010). Why partnership working doesn't work. *Public Management Review.* **12** (6), 811–28.

Dowling, B., Powell, M. & Glendinning, C. (2004). Conceptualising successful partnerships. *Health and Social Care in the Community.* **12** (4), 309–14.

Ferlie, E., Fitzgerald, L., McGivern, G., Dopson, S. & Bennet, C. (2013). *Making Wicked Problems Governable? The Case of Managed Networks in Health Care.* Oxford: Oxford University Press.

Furber, C. & Thomson, A. (2010). The power of language: a secondary analysis of a qualitative study exploring English midwives' support of mothers' baby-feeding practice. *Midwifery.* **26** (2), 232–40.

Glasby, J. & Dickinson, H. (2014). *Partnership working in health and social care*. Bristol: Policy Press.

Glasby, J., Dickinson, H. & Miller, R. (2011). Partnership working in England – where we are now and where we've come from. *International Journal of Integrated Care.* **11**, 1–8.

Glendinning, C., Powell, M. & Rummery, K. (2002). *Partnerships, New Labour and the Governance of Welfare.* Bristol: Policy Press.

Greenwood, E. (1957). Attributes of a profession. *Social Work.* **2** (3), 44–55.

Hall, P. (2005). Interprofessional teamwork: Professional cultures as barriers. *Journal of Interprofessional Care.* **1**, 188–96.

Hansard (1997). *Hansard Debates 9 Dec 1997: Column 796.* Available from: http://www.publications.parliament.uk/pa/cm199798/cmhansrd/vo971209/debtext/71209-05.htm (last accessed: 13. 12.2016).

Hudson, B. (2010). The Three Ps in the NHS White Paper: Partnership, Privatisation and Predation: Which way will it go and does it matter? *Journal of Integrated Care.* **18** (5), 15–24.

Hudson, B. (2002). Interprofessionality in health and social care: the Achilles' heel of partnership? *Journal of Interprofessional Care.* **16** (1), 7–17.

Humphries, R. & Wenzel, L (2015). *Options for Integrated Commissioning.* London: The King's Fund.

Hunter, D.J. & Perkins, Neil (2014). *Partnership working in public health.* Bristol: Policy Press.

Huxham, C. & Vangen, S. (2005). *Managing to collaborate: The theory and practice of collaborative advantage.* London: Routledge.

Lester, H., Birchwood, M., Tait, L., Shah, S., England, E. & Smith, J. (2008). Barriers and facilitators to partnership working between Early Intervention Services and the voluntary and community sector. *Health and Social Care in the Community.* **16** (5), 493–500.

Loxely, A. (1997). *Collaboration in Health and Welfare.* London: Jessica Kingsley.

Lukes, S. (2005). *Power – a radical view.* 2nd edn. London: Macmillan.

Malin, N. (2000). *Professionalism, boundaries and the workplace.* London: Routledge.

Petch, A., Cook, A. & Miller, E. (2013). Partnership working and outcomes: do health and social care partnerships deliver for users and carers? *Health and Social Care in the Community.* **21** (6), 623–33.

Rummery, K. (2009). Healthy partnerships, healthy citizens? An international review of partnerships in health and social care and patient/user outcomes. *Social Services and Medicine.* **69**, 1797–1804.

Scottish Government (2015). *Public Bodies (Joint Working) (Scotland) Act.* http://www.gov.scot/Topics/Health/Policy/Adult-Health-SocialCare-Integration/About-the-Bill (last accessed 14.3.2016).

Tritter, J. & McCallum, A. (2006). The snakes and ladders of user involvement: Moving beyond Arnstein. *Health Policy.* **76** (2), 156–68.

Welsh Government (2015). *Social Services and Well-Being (Wales) Act 2014 Part 9 Statutory Guidance (Partnership Arrangements).* http://gov.wales/docs/dhss/publications/151218part9en.pdf (last accessed 13.12.2016).

Wildridge, V., Childs, S., Cawthra, L. & Madge, B. (2004). How to create successful partnerships – a review of the literature. *Health Information and Libraries Journal.* **21**, 3–19.

Willis, E. (2006). Taking stock of medical dominance. *Health Sociology Review.* **15** (5), 421–31.

Chapter 7

Communication in the digital age

Fiona Fraser and Katrina Bannigan

Learning outcomes
By the end of this chapter you will be able to:
- Differentiate the various forms of communication used by health and social care professionals
- Reflect on whom you communicate with in a professional context
- Recognise the opportunities and challenges presented by social media when working as a health and social care professional
- Explain the expectations placed upon health and social care professionals in terms of appropriate and effective communication

What is communication?

Competence in communication is about being able to use verbal, non-verbal, written, visual and digital skills to convey information or to express opinions. Communication can therefore come in many forms and usually involves interaction with others. The most common types of communication include written or spoken communication, verbal or non-verbal, and formal or informal.

Written or spoken communication
Both these forms of communication involve the use of words but one is communicated visually (e.g. through telephone messages, emails or word-processed documents on a computer) and the other aurally.

Verbal or non-verbal
Whilst a person hears verbal communication if they can see the person who is communicating with them (e.g. if they are speaking face-to-face or using skype), what is

communicated will be augmented by visual information, such as facial expressions, body language and gestures. This additional visual information (non-verbal communication) may change the sense of the words to something slightly different from what they would have meant if they had only been heard. This is what is meant by the expression 'it's the way you said it'.

Formal or informal

This distinction is about the style of communication and it is usually shaped by context. Formal communication is the main form of communication used by health and social care professionals when they are at work. It is characterised by a formal tone, a lack of slang, and following rules, such as the correct use of grammar and/or etiquette (e.g. waiting to be invited to speak by the chair, before speaking in a meeting). Informal communication is generally used outside work and is characterised by a relaxed tone and the use of slang. The usual rules of conversation (e.g. turn-taking) are less likely to be observed. However, there are no hard and fast rules about when to use formal and informal communication. For instance, a professional outside work, speaking to their grandmother, may use formal communication. Another professional at work may choose to be informal in their communication because there is a sense of what is needed, e.g. making a joke to lighten the mood. It takes skill to judge which style is appropriate for the situation and it needs to be judged very carefully. For example, an inopportune joke may backfire and worsen a situation.

Health and social care professionals need to be adept at all forms of communication because good communication is essential for building rapport and forming positive therapeutic relationships with patients (Persaud 2005, Sims 2014). This chapter will refer to the people health and social care professionals work with as patients although it is acknowledged that other terms (such as service user or client) may better suit some settings. Communication is a highly skilled activity that involves rudimentary skills, such as listening, being approachable and being attentive, and more complex skills such as empathy, congruence and acceptance (Bonham 2004). Depending on the field they work in, health and social care professionals may also need to learn alternative forms of communication, such as sign language or visual communication. For example, professionals working with people with learning disabilities may need to use Makaton (a form of communication that uses signs and symbols).

The value of good communication goes beyond the patient–professional relationship; it also has an impact on patient outcome (Persaud 2005, Brown *et al.* 2006). Good communication is perceived as being integral to the quality of care which is why it is included in the 6Cs – care, compassion, courage, communication, commitment and competence (Stephenson 2014). The 6Cs were originally the core nursing values but have been rolled out to all staff working in the NHS in England to characterise 'Our Culture of Compassionate Care' (NHS 2012a). Communication is integral to quality of care partly due to the sheer variety of people a health and social care professional has to communicate with.

Who do we communicate with?

Health and social care professionals communicate with a wide range of people, including patients, their families and carers, colleagues (both within and outside the team) and other agencies and organisations.

Patients

When communicating with a patient we need to take into account, and respect, the fact that their cultural background will shape their beliefs and customs related to communication; this includes choosing the language they wish to communicate with. The setting will also influence communication. For example, in an acute mental health setting a patient may be disorientated, confused and frightened by being in an unfamiliar place and may therefore find it difficult to retain information. This will require a different approach to communication, i.e. repeating information many times, orientating the patient to their surroundings, and providing reassurance (Sims 2014), which may not be appropriate when meeting a patient in their own home or in a community setting. For a person with a learning disability, it may be necessary to establish how best to communicate with them before starting to work with them (Goodman & Wright 2014). Working with patients involves decision-making, regardless of setting, and this should be shared decision-making if we aspire to our stated aim of making 'no decision about me without me' (NHS 2012b).

Successful decision-making depends on good communication (Elwyn *et al.* 2012). Shared decision-making involves patients being listened to and having their views and opinions respected. According to Elwyn *et al.* (2012), they need:

- sufficient information presented in jargon-free language
- the opportunity to discuss their options
- support in the process of deliberation.

Face-to-face communication is still commonly used but other means of communicating with patients are increasingly being used, such as telephone consultation. With non-face-to-face forms, the lack of visual cues (Car *et al.* 2004) requires professionals to adopt different communication strategies, such as framing questions to increase patient disclosure and responding to emotional cues (Shaw *et al.* 2013) in order to foster strong therapeutic relationships.

Carers

Professionals are likely to benefit from communicating with carers because they are the family members, partners or friends who provide informal support to patients (Small *et al.* 2010). However, it is very important to secure a patient's consent before speaking to anyone else about their care. The patient may not wish you to speak to, or involve, their carer in a current episode of care and their wishes should be respected (Donskoy *et al.* 2014). Nonetheless, 'it is important to remember that it is still possible to listen to a carer's point of view and experience without breaching confidentiality. This can be done by listening but not providing any information' (Sims 2014, p. 349). If permission to involve a carer is given, it is important to recognise the complexity of the patient–carer relationship which adds another dynamic to the communication process and may add bias to information given. The carer may also need support or education, which will require the health and social care professional to use different communication skills, e.g. facilitating a group discussion in a carers' support group.

Colleagues in our team(s)

Team working is central to the delivery of health and social care, and good communication contributes to good team dynamics. This is why the 6Cs refer to the workplace and the benefits of good communication for staff as well as patients (NHS 2012a). To communicate well with your team, you need to be inclusive, open and collaborative in your communication style (Apker *et al.* 2006). Your colleagues need to be kept up to date about your work with patients, and you need to listen to their views about the patient's progress. You also need to be prepared to liaise and negotiate with colleagues, particularly regarding the organisation of care to prevent duplication or over-burdening the patient (e.g. by numerous colleagues asking the patient for the same information). Although most communication between team members will be verbal, the information will also be written in patient notes and reports. To facilitate communication, documentation should be well written – not only in terms of content but good grammar and presentation, which will also show colleagues your professionalism and attention to detail. Written documentation must also conform to the standards of conduct, performance and ethics relevant to your particular profession.

Colleagues outside your team(s)

We communicate with the wider community of health and social care professionals to create, share or exchange information. For example, we make referrals to outside agencies such as third sector bodies or wider public sector organisations like the police or liaise with schools to provide support for children to remain in mainstream education. All forms of communication are used: email, written documents, face-to-face meetings and telephone calls; in each episode of communication confidentiality should not be breached.

It is probably with colleagues outside our teams that we are most likely to use social media for communication; indeed it has been widely promoted for this purpose (Bannigan 2016). We can communicate with the widest possible audiences of health and social care professionals through different programmes or platforms such as Facebook, Instagram, Twitter and YouTube. The ubiquitous nature of social media means that all health and social care professionals have a social media profile, regardless of whether they actively engage in social media themselves. As such, we have a professional duty to manage our profile (Burgess & Humphries 2015) and, because social media often bridges both our professional and social lives, it is critical to consider the professional implications of using social media (see below).

Other agencies

Health and social care professionals often need to communicate with third parties, e.g. providing reports to solicitors as expert witnesses or liaising with a residential home about someone's care needs. When a health and social care professional does this, the patient expects that the information they have disclosed will be treated confidentially and will only be shared when and with whom it has been explicitly agreed (Beighton & Collins 2014). Inaccurate communication (e.g. illegible handwriting, ambiguous abbreviations or mishearing instructions) can result in adverse events so it is imperative that all communication with other agencies is correct, with no room for misinterpretation (Koczmara *et al.* 2006).

This section has hinted at how communication is evolving due to changes in technology in wider society, and this process of evolution is likely to continue. This subject is further explored below.

The changing context of communication

In the past, health and social care professionals worked and communicated in a comparatively localised context. On occasions there may have been opportunities to interact at a broader level by attending a conference or meeting. However, communication was largely limited to face-to-face interactions or via the telephone or fax. However, with the introduction of the Internet, and then social media, a whole new range of communication channels have evolved. Our professional networks are often global. Best practice can be shared around the world and reach vast audiences in a matter of minutes. For example, 'Online social networks such as Facebook offer a fast and easily accessible online space to form communities of practice while also enabling us to work towards enhancing public awareness of … [our professions]' (Kashani *et al.* 2010, p.22). Although the traditional forms of communication still play a large part in our everyday lives, the technology evolution is experienced on a daily basis (Bargh & McKenna 2004).

How can we define social media?

Social media may be defined as 'a form of interaction by which people create, share, exchange and comment among themselves within a virtual (online) community or network' (Foster 2013, p.98). Between January and March 2015, 86% of adults (44.7 million) in the UK had used the Internet in the last 3 months (Office of National Statistics 2015). In the same year Ofcom, the regulator and competitions authority for the UK communications industry, published figures suggesting that 72% of all Internet users have a social media profile.

Technology has not only become part of the lives of health and social care professionals; our patients are also becoming more technology savvy. Technology is now part of the fabric of everyday life, through the use of online banking, social networking, computer games and online education (Brown 2011). Many applications of social media facilitate our patients' independence – for example, being able to shop online and have groceries delivered. Social media and the Internet have also increased opportunities for patients to research their health and potential treatment options (Fox 2011). This can include the use of discussion forums as well as blogs to chronicle their progress and share their experiences. NHS Choices (2015) are currently reviewing a range of health-related smartphone applications, having launched the 'Health App Library' in 2013, bringing medical knowledge/advice to people via their smartphones. This in turn could potentially decrease the burden on primary health care services.

Reflective questions

- How could you use technology in your own area of professional practice?
- Specifically, could technology be used to enhance communication in your workplace? If so, in what ways?

Types of social media

There are various different types of social media that are used for different purposes. Ventola (2014) loosely categorises them as social and professional networking, media sharing, content production, knowledge/information aggregation and virtual reality/gaming environments.

Social networking (e.g. Facebook, Myspace, Google+)

These are used primarily for social reasons, such as communicating with friends, sharing memories, photographs and opinions. However, professional bodies such as the Health and Care Professions Council (see https://www.facebook.com/hcpcuk) maintain an active Facebook page as a means to communicate with allied health professionals, to share news and common points of interest with its registrants.

Professional networking (e.g. LinkedIn, Research Gate)
Professional networking groups, such as LinkedIn, provide a space to post an online version of your Curriculum Vitae, along with space to engage in a wide range of discussion groups. For example, the Mental Health Networking Group identify themselves on LinkedIn as a group for people working in mental health who would like to expand their network and reach out to others, to exchange ideas, expertise and best practice (LinkedIn 2016).

Media sharing (e.g. YouTube, Flickr, Instagram, Pinterest)
Media sharing provides users with an opportunity to curate their own media in the form of collections of videos or images. Many charities post public awareness videos on YouTube, such as the Alzheimer's disease Society (see https://www.youtube.com/user/AlzheimersSociety).

Content production (e.g. blogs such as Tumblr and Blogger and microblogs like Twitter)
Communities such as @WeNurses, @WeMidwives and @weAHPs, host chats on Twitter to support best practice in health and social care (see http://www.wecommunities.org/about).

Knowledge/information aggregation (e.g. Wikipedia)
Although widely acknowledged not to be an appropriate source for academic assignments (Harvard 2016), Wikipedia is useful when seeking an overview on a specific topic. For example, occupational therapy has a robust Wikipedia entry (see https://en.wikipedia.org/wiki/Occupational therapy) that charts its development as a profession.

Virtual reality and gaming environments (e.g. Second Life)
Virtual reality sites, like Second Life, allow users to create virtual avatars of themselves and interact within a simulated 3D context. Social media of this type has real potential in terms of student education and it has been used with student nurses to enable them develop/practise professional skills within a 'safe' environment (Patterson *et al.* 2015).

The content of our communication
Regardless of the diverse and complex ways in which health and social care professionals can communicate, the content of our communication is essentially the same, e.g. supporting decision-making, providing education, reporting and sharing bad news. Being clear and effective, regardless of the form or content of communication, is an essential requirement for all health and social care professionals (Hargie 2011). To take giving bad news as an illustrative example, 'bad news' is any information which adversely or seriously affects an individual's view of their future (Buckman 1992). Breaking bad news is a challenging aspect of being a health or social care professional and Baile *et al.* (2000) set out the SPIKES protocol as a method of breaking down the areas that need consideration when presenting bad news. Originally developed for the field of oncology, the process can be applied to other situations:

- **S (setting)**: Consider the environment in which the conversation is going to take place. For instance, a noisy corridor or an open-plan office will be less appropriate than a quiet room.
- **P (perspective)**: As the 'news breaker', you will need to be prepared. Therefore it is useful to consider the other person's perspective before and during the conversation. Ask questions and ensure they follow the information that you are share.
- **I (invitation)**: Give the individual an opportunity to ask questions. Seek clarity about how they want the information to be presented.
- **K (knowledge)**: Consider the timing and flow of the information that you are providing. Avoid jargon and inaccessible language.
- **E (emotions)**: Understand that the individual may need to express their emotions and try to empathise with their situation.
- **S (strategy and summary)**: Provide the individual with an overview of the situation and give them information about what is going to happen next.

The SPIKES protocol is an example of how communication skills can be honed. As well as being aware of the need to be skilled communicators, registered health and social care professionals, need to be mindful that our communication and conduct outside work can also come under scrutiny (Health and Care Professions Council 2015, Nursing and Midwifery Council 2015, General Medical Council 2013).

Social media and professionalism

Social media provides many opportunities for communication with wide and varied audiences but it must be harnessed in a professional manner. The various forms of social media, increasingly accessible via smartphones, have unfortunately amplified the potential for lapses in professional judgement (Gholami-Kordkheili *et al.* 2013). For those working within a regulated health/social care profession, the inappropriate use of social media can lead to disciplinary action. Moreover, the implications of any misuse can have lasting repercussions for the individual's career and professional standing. For example, the Health and Care Professions Council make public (via their website) the details of the hearings they hold when allegations are made against a registrant.

Reflective questions
- Who do you communicate with when using social media?
- Is social media an appropriate forum to communicate with patients?
- If yes, in what context?

Professional expectations

Regulators such as the Health and Care Professions Council (HCPC), the Nursing and Midwifery Council (NMC) and the General Medical Council (GMC) all set out expectations for their registrants in terms of communication (HCPC 2015, NMC 2015, GMC 2013). Failure to meet these expectations can potentially lead to professionals being removed from the register and therefore no longer being able to practise within their chosen field. It is therefore vital for us to remain cognisant of our how our professional and personal communication can be interpreted as well as misinterpreted.

Online communication has increased the potential for professional dialogue to be 'lost in translation', as we have no control over how other people will interpret our emails or tweets, especially if read out of context (Kruger *et al.* 2005). Without the ability to convey emotion and variation in tone, our email communication is 'one-dimensional'. In addition, the accessibility of email means we have no control over the time and situation the reader finds themselves in when they engage with our message. However, regulators are aware that social media is now part of registrants' personal and professional lives (Foster 2013) and have started to provide guidelines to help clarify their expectations (HCPC 2015, NMC 2016, GMC 2013). These highlight how ethical considerations such as maintaining confidentiality, conflicts of interest, privacy and the sharing of personal information all need to be considered (Moorhead *et al.* 2013).

Nonetheless, with mature handling, social media can be helpful in broadening the range of communications typically available to health and social care professionals. McNab (2009) suggests that, rather than showing concern about social media, health professionals need to use it to be present in sometimes global conversations, to pass on information and also to add value to the discussion and help correct rumours or misinformation. This is particularly important in view of the fact that the 'virtual world' does not filter out bad-quality information (Harvard 2016). For example, a dietitian can use a blog or Twitter to dispel myths about dieting and certain 'super foods' that are being promoted by the mass media.

Conclusion

Communication has a strong impact on the therapeutic relationship and outcome of care. It is also a skill that can be learnt; communication skills can always be improved, no matter how experienced we are as health and social care professionals. Being aware of the different types of communication and who they may be directed at, as explored in this chapter, is a useful exercise when reflecting on and developing our communication skills. In addition, harnessing social media to communicate with a wider audience can help us develop us as digital leaders (Hunter 2013). New graduate practitioners have the opportunity to make the transition into practice with a 'global support network', whilst established health and social care professionals have the ability to refresh and extend their professional networks.

This chapter has also explored the challenges associated with social media which can potentially blur the boundaries between our professional and personal lives. However, with effective and mature handling of issues around privacy, confidentiality and sensitive information, social media can enhance our communication on a local, national and global scale. As health and social care professionals, who are lifelong learners, communication is a skill we should invest in developing throughout our careers. After all, as this chapter has demonstrated, 'Communication skills by definition never stand still; we are always learning, and are forever being enriched by new developments, new challenges and new opportunities' (Moss 2015, p.xiii).

Reflective questions

- Think about who you communicate with and the different methods of communication that you use.
- What safeguards do you employ to ensure that you stay within professional boundaries?

References

Apker, J., Propp, K.M., Zabava-Ford, W.S. & Hofmeister, N. (2006). Collaboration, credibility, compassion, and coordination: Professional nurse communication skill sets in health care team interactions. *Journal of Professional Nursing.* **22** (3), 180–89.

Arora, A., McNab, M.A., Lewis, M.W., Hilton, G., Blinkhorn, A.S. & Schwarz, E. (2012). 'I can't relate it to teeth': A qualitative approach to evaluate oral health education materials for preschool children in New South Wales, Australia. *International Journal of Paediatric Dentistry.* **22** (4), 302–309.

Baile, W.F., Buckman, R., Lenzi, R., Glober, G., Beale, E.A. & Kudelka, A.P. (2000). SPIKES – A six step, protocol for delivering bad news: application to the patient with cancer. *The Oncologist.* **5**, 302–11.

Bakurst, K. (2011). *How has social media changed the way newsrooms work?* http://www.bbc.co.uk/blogs/theeditors/2011/09/ibc_in_amsterdam.html (last accessed 15.3.2016).

Bannigan, K. (2016). How effective is your social media profile? *Occupational Therapy News.* **24** (1), 24–25.

Bargh, J.A. & McKenna, K.Y.A. (2004). The internet and social life. *Annual Review of Psychology.* **55** (1), 573–90.

Beighton, C. & Collins, B. (2014). 'Professional Accountability' in W. Bryant, J. Fieldhouse & K. Bannigan (eds) *Creek's Occupational Therapy and Mental Health.* 5th edn. Edinburgh: Churchill Livingstone.

Bonham, P. (2004). *Communicating as a Mental Health Carer.* Cheltenham: Nelson Thornes.

Brown, B., Crawford, P. & Carter, R. (2006). *Evidence-based Health Communication.* Maidenhead: Open University Press.

Brown, E. (2011). Are you a digital native or a digital immigrant? Being client centred in the digital era. *British Journal of Occupational Therapy.* **74** (7), 313.

Buckman, R. (1992). *Breaking Bad News: A Guide for Health Care Professionals*. Baltimore: Johns Hopkins University Press.

Burgess, S. & Humphries, R. (2015). Developing an e-presence within the profession. *Occupational Therapy News*. **23** (1), 22–23.

Car, J., Freeman, G.K., Partridge, M.R. & Sheikh, A. (2004). Improving quality and safety of telephone based delivery of care: teaching telephone consultation skills. *Quality and Safety in Health Care*. **13**, 2–3.

Donskoy, A.L., Stevens, R. & Bryant, W. (2014). 'Perspectives on using and providing services' in W. Bryant, J. Fieldhouse & K. Bannigan (eds) *Creek's Occupational Therapy and Mental Health*. 5th edn. Edinburgh: Churchill Livingstone.

Elwyn, G., Frosch, D., Thomson, R., Joseph-Williams, N., Lloyd, A., Kinnersley, P., Cording, E., Tomson, D., Dodd, C., Rollnick, S., Edwards, A. & Barry, M. (2012). Shared decision making: a model for clinical practice. *Journal of General Internal Medicine*. **27** (10), 1361–67.

Foster, J. (2013). Social media. *Journal of the Irish Dental Association*. **59** (2), 98–99.

Fox, S. (2011) *Peer-to-peer healthcare. Pew Internet & American Life Project*. http://pewinternet.org/Reports/2011/P2PHealthcare.aspx (last accessed 20.3.2016).

General Medical Council (GMC) (2013). *Good Medical Practice*. London: GMC.

Gholami-Kordkheili, F., Wild, V. & Strech, D. (2013). The impact of social media on medical professionalism: a systematic qualitative review of challenges and opportunities. *Journal of Medical Internet Research*. **15** (8), 184.

Goodman, J. & Wright, W. (2014). 'Learning disabilities' in W. Bryant, J. Fieldhouse & K. Bannigan (eds) *Creek's Occupational Therapy and Mental Health*. 5th edn. Edinburgh: Churchill Livingstone.

Hargie, O. (2011). *Skilled interpersonal communication, research, theory and practice*. 5th edn. East Sussex: Routledge.

Harvard (2016). *What's Wrong with Wikipedia? Harvard Guide to Using Sources*. http://actioncivics.scoe.net/pdf/Harvard-Guide-to-Using-Sources.pdf (last accessed 30.9.2017).

Health and Care Professions Council (HCPC) (2015). *Standards of conduct, performance and ethics*. London: HCPC.

Hunter, E.P. (2013). The Elizabeth Casson Memorial Lecture 2013: Transformational Leadership in Occupational Therapy – Delivering Change through Conversations. *British Journal of Occupational Therapy*. **76** (8), 346–54.

Kashani, R., Burwash, S. & Hamiliton, A. (2010). To be or not be on Facebook: That is the question. *Occupational Therapy Now*. **21** (6), 19–22.

Koczmara, C., Jelincic, V. & Perri, D. (2006). Communication of medication orders by telephone – 'Writing it right'. *Dynamics*. **17** (1), 20–24.

Kruger, J., Epley, N., Parker, J. & Ng, Z. (2005). Egocentrism over E-mail: Can we communicate as well as we think? *Journal of Personality and Social Psychology*. **89** (6), 925–36.

LinkedIn (2016). *Mental Health Networking*. https://www.linkedin.com/groups/141502/profile (last accessed: 16.12.2016).

McCrindle, M. (2006). *New generations at work: attracting, recruiting, retaining, and training generation Y*. http://mccrindle.com.au/resources/whitepapers/McCrindle-Research_New-Generations-At-Work-attracting-recruiting-retaining-training-generation-y.pdf (last accessed 30.9.2017).

McNab, C. (2009). What social media offers to health professionals and citizens. *Bulletin of the World Health Organization*. **87** (8), 566.

Moorhead, S.A., Hazlett, D.E., Harrison, L., Carroll, J.K., Irwin, A. & Hoving, C. (2013). A New Dimension of Health Care: Systematic Review of the Uses, Benefits, and Limitations of Social Media for Health Communication. *Journal of Medical Internet Research* **15** (4), 85.

Moss, B. (2015). *Communication Skills in Health and Social Care*. 3rd edn. London: Sage.

NHS (2012a). *Our Culture of Compassionate Care.* https://www.ardengemcsu.nhs.uk/files/3914/8596/3150/A15_-_6c-visual.pdf (last accessed 30.8.2017).

NHS (2012b). *Liberating the NHS: No decision about me, without me.* https://www.gov.uk/government/uploads/system/uploads/attachment_data/file/216980/Liberating-the-NHS-No-decision-about-me-without-me-Government-response.pdf (last accessed 5.6.2016).

NHS Choices (2015). *Health Apps Library.* http://www.nhs.uk/pages/healthappslibrary.aspx (last accessed 20.3.2016).

Nursing and Midwifery Council (NMC) (2015). *The Code. Professional Standards of Practice and behaviour for nurses and midwives.* London: NMC.

Nursing and Midwifery Council (NMC) (2016). *Guidance on using social media responsibly.* https://www.nmc.org.uk/standards/guidance/social-media-guidance (last accessed 5.6.2016).

Ofcom (2015). *The Communications Market.* http://stakeholders.ofcom.org.uk/market-data-research/market-data/communications-market-reports/cmr15 (last accessed 13.3.2016).

Office of National Statistics (2015). *Statistical bulletin: Internet users: 2015.* http://www.ons.gov.uk/businessindustryandtrade/itandinternetindustry/bulletins/internetusers/2015 (last accessed 13.3.2016).

Patterson, B.J., Tilton, K.J., Jone, T. & Hoglund, B.A. (2015). Non-acute care, virtual stimulation; preparing students to provide chronic illness care. *Nurse Education Perspectives.* **36** (6), 394–95.

Persaud, R. (2005). How to improve communication with patients. *British Medical Journal Career Focus.* **2**, 136–37.

Prensky, M. (2001). Digital Natives, Digital Immigrants. *On the Horizon.* MCB University Press. **9** (5), 1–6.

Shaw, J., Young, J., Butow, P., Chambers, S., O'Brien, L. & Solomon, M., (2013). Delivery of telephone-based supportive care to people with cancer: An analysis of cancer helpline operator and cancer nurse communication. *Patient Education and Counseling.* **93** (3), 444–50.

Sims, K.L. (2014). 'The Acute Setting' in W. Bryant, J. Fieldhouse & K. Bannigan (eds) *Creek's Occupational Therapy and Mental Health.* 5th edn. Edinburgh: Churchill Livingstone.

Stephenson, J. (2014). *NHS England to roll out '6Cs' nursing values to all health service staff.* http://www.nursingtimes.net/roles/nurse-managers/exclusive-6cs-nursing-values-to-be-rolled-outto-all-nhs-staff/5070102.fullarticle (last accessed 21.2.2016).

Ventola, C.L. (2014). Social media and health care professionals: benefits, risks, and best practices. *Pharmacy and Therapeutics.* **39** (7), 491–520.

Section 3
Quality in practice

Introduction
by Steven W. Whitcombe

In health and social care, 'quality' is paramount and so the quality of your practice should always be your central concern. As you 'move through' your career, you will encounter various policies, initiatives and political drivers that focus on the issue of quality. Having read this section of the book, you will see that policies relating to quality may have a different perspective depending on, for example, the health and social care needs of a particular local population. Nevertheless, 'quality' as a construct remains the same and, as professionals, we have a duty to ensure that our practice is safe, effective, evidence-based and meets the needs of our service users.

Chapter 8 focuses on the political and legal interface with professional practice. In order to practise effectively, the author of this chapter argues that health and social care practitioners need to have an understanding of the policy-making and legislative process and its influence on driving quality initiatives. This chapter considers how legislative frameworks relating to quality differ across the devolved nations of the United Kingdom. It also discusses the measures that professional organisations use to assess the quality of health and social care practice. These can vary according to where you live and work in the United Kingdom – for example, the Care Quality Commission in England, as opposed to the Care Inspectorate in Scotland. This chapter concludes by asking you to reflect on how you can ensure the quality of your practice.

Chapter 9 addresses the challenges of maintaining quality in health and social care in a climate of fiscal constraint. Health and social care practitioners are often required to do more and provide better services with less money and fewer resources. This chapter considers how care services are commissioned in the United Kingdom and how market forces affect the provision of health and social care. The chapter encourages you to think about different ways of delivering quality services and to reflect on how you can be innovative and entrepreneurial in your own practice.

Finally, Chapter 10 discusses the role of research and its relationship with evidence-based practice. It begins with an overview of different research traditions and methodologies and looks at how these can be applied to practice. All health and social care professionals should be consumers of research but this chapter goes further and offers suggestions on how you can take a more active research role in the workplace or even consider research as a career.

In order to get the most from these chapters, we ask that you really engage with and reflect on the questions and practical exercises you will find in them. It is only through an honest and meaningful exploration of your own beliefs and values that the full benefit of this reading will be experienced.

Chapter 8
The political and legal interface with professional practice

Heather Hunter

Learning outcomes
By the end of this chapter you will be able to:
- Explain how government policy and laws affect the health and social care sector and the relevance of laws and policy for the health care practitioner
- Recognise how 'a bill' becomes an act of parliament
- Explain how policies and acts differ between the devolved nations of the United Kingdom
- Reflect on the role of professional and regulatory bodies in monitoring health and social care practice.

Background
Due to a rise in life expectancy, coupled with decreasing resources, the health and social care sector is a significant area for political parties hoping to gain political security by 'solving' the issue of increasing demand on services. Equally, mistakes in hospitals such as Bristol Royal Infirmary where the deaths of 29 babies undergoing heart surgery were investigated (Kennedy Report 2010), and the implications of poor management and leadership leading to significant failure in caring for patients, as occurred at the Mid Staffordshire Foundation Trust (Francis Report 2013), can affect the policies that government introduce, so that lessons are 'seen to be learned' and recommendations are put into practice (see also Section 4 of this book). Rhetoric from government ministers and other commentators claim that this is accomplished via a number of strategies: the publication of policy documents, such as the NHS *Five Year Forward View* (Department of Health 2014); legislation through Acts of Parliament, e.g. Health and Social Care Act

(Department of Health 2013) and the introduction of an updated NHS *Constitution for England* in 2015.

Moreover, the government's decision to devolve power has led to the UK Parliament handing over some powers to other countries' parliaments, including Scotland, Wales and Northern Ireland. These devolved powers include responsibility for health, education, local government and the environment. This has led to different countries directing resources in different ways, to meet the differing needs of their populations, further complicating the health care arena for future and current practitioners who may work in the different countries. As part of this process, the government assemblies in Scotland, Wales and Northern Ireland have tackled their different health care needs with different policies: for example, the '1000 lives plus' campaign (NHS Public Health Wales 2012) focuses on improving the health and safety of patients with an emphasis on enhanced recovery from surgery and a reduction in errors in patient identification and falls. Meanwhile, Scotland has introduced the National Musculoskeletal Advice and Triage Service (NHS Scotland) for adults with musculoskeletal problems. So, rather than attending outpatient departments, which may be sparsely located due to the geographical remoteness and low population in some areas of Scotland, patients can access advice and support over the phone.

Specific scandals, such as the death of 'Baby P' at the hands of his mother and her boyfriend, led to the second Laming Report (2009); and the public inquiry into poor standards of patient care at the Mid Staffordshire NHS Foundation Trust (Francis Report 2013) has led to calls for more effective monitoring by the Care Quality Commission as well as regulatory bodies such as the Health and Care Professions Council (HCPC) and the Nursing and Midwifery Council (NMC) to maintain standards that will safeguard and protect the public.

Health care practitioners therefore need to be aware of the political and legal aspects of health care to ensure that they practise safely, efficaciously and with due regard to the law. This chapter introduces health care practitioners to the stages that a bill goes through before it is given royal assent and introduced into law as an act. This will be outlined using current examples of UK legislation such as the Health and Social Care Act (2013) which detailed significant changes to commissioning of services and brought public health under the auspices of the NHS. We will also consider policy drivers such as the NHS *Five Year Forward View* (2014), which was designed to improve patient care by preventing ill health and engaging communities with regard to delivery of health services. All health care practitioners entering health service employment will be asked to commit to the 'Values Based Behaviour' set out in the *NHS Constitution* (2015), which includes the values: working together for patients; respect and dignity; commitment to quality care; compassion; improving lives; and everyone counts.

This chapter will introduce health care practitioners to how health care policy is implemented and how it shapes and develops practice nationally and locally, using examples of particular acts and policy documents. It will then review the roles of the professional and regulatory bodies of the allied health professions as well as the organisations that monitor safety and quality.

Green and white papers and acts of parliament

Green and white papers are policy documents that are produced by relevant government departments to explain their proposals for future legislation. A green paper is a consultative document which allows interested parties (both within and outside parliament) to give feedback on each policy or legislative proposal. It is designed to facilitate debate and discussion and each proposal usually includes several alternatives which are discussed before a final decision on the best policy is made. It is worth noting that there can be more than one consultation and that this can be quite a long process, resulting in significant changes and at times a 'watering down' and/or refining of the initial proposals.

At the state opening of parliament, the monarch sets out the government's agenda for the coming session (normally 12 months, from November), and outlines the government's proposed policies and legislation. While the monarch reads out the speech, the content is entirely written by the government and approved by the cabinet and the monarch is only there in a ceremonial capacity. The content of the speech indicates what will be discussed and formally agreed by both houses of parliament (i.e. the House of Commons and the House of Lords) and what will end up as law. The speech also mentions policies that set a direction which are not enforceable by law, for example, the *Five Year Forward View* (Department of Health 2014).

Ideas for changes in the law are either set out as a green or a white paper. A white paper is more detailed than a green paper and is shaped by the government department from which it stems. The white paper is then published as a command paper by the relevant government department (e.g. the Department of Health), which sets out their proposals for future legislation. Interested or affected groups can provide feedback and final changes can be made: again, this can be quite a lengthy process. These final changes are either formulated into a bill proposing a new law, or as a proposal to change an existing law.

A bill is formally presented to parliament and the first stage of a bill's passage through the House of Commons (usually a formality) takes place without debate. This is known as the first reading. The next stage is the second reading, which is the first opportunity that members of parliament (MPs) have to debate the general principles of the bill. At the second reading, the government minister or spokesperson for the bill opens the debate, which is subsequently responded to by the 'official opposition'. At the end of the debate, the Commons decides whether the bill should be given its second reading by voting, meaning it can proceed to the next stage – the committee stage.

If passed, the bill is dealt with in a 'public bill committee', which is a subsection of cross-party MPs (though there is always a government majority). The number of members of a public bill committee ranges from a minimum of 16 to a maximum of 50. At this stage, each clause (part) and any amendments (proposals for change) to the bill are discussed and voted on by the committee. Every clause is either agreed to, changed or removed, and the committee is able to take evidence from experts and interest groups to assist them with this process. Once the committee stage is finished, the bill returns to the floor of the House of Commons for its report stage, where the amended bill can be debated by the whole House, with further amendments proposed. All MPs may speak and vote on the bill and lengthy or complex bills may take several days to proceed.

The report stage is normally followed by debate on the bill's third reading, which is the final chance for the Commons to debate the content of the bill. Such debate is usually short and limited to what is actually *in* the bill, rather than, as at the second reading, what might have been included. Amendments cannot be made at this stage. At the end of the debate, the House votes on whether to approve the third reading of the bill. If the bill is passed, it will enter the House of Lords for its first reading and the process is repeated. When a bill has passed through the third reading in both Houses of Parliament, it is returned to the first house (where it started) for the second house's amendments to be considered. This may result in the bill going backwards and forwards between both houses, but both houses must agree to the exact wording of the bill. Once the Commons and the Lords agree the final version of the bill, it can receive royal assent by the reigning monarch; then it will become an Act of Parliament, which is enforced in all areas of the UK where applicable.

A recent example of a white paper being transformed into legislation was the introduction of 'Equity and Excellence: Liberating the NHS' white paper, which was published under the government coalition in July 2010, but only passed into law as the Health and Social Care Act (Department of Health 2013).

The Health and Social Care Act (2013) was one of the biggest changes in the health care system for a considerable time and was introduced in a context of significant financial challenges. Some of the major changes included: establishing an independent NHS board to allocate resources; increased GP powers to commission services; cuts to the number of health bodies including abolishing Primary Care Trust and Strategic

Health Authorities. Further changes include creating a joint budget for health and social care, controlled by GP commissioners who are given responsibility for purchasing services based on a local needs assessment. These developments are aimed at giving patients more of a voice and creating greater local accountability, while reducing costs through the pooling of budgets. Another key aspect of the Health and Social Care Act (2013) was the introduction of competition for the provision of services. This resulted in the process of identifying any qualified provider who would be able to bid to deliver the service. Arguably, competition was seen as a way of reducing costs for services. These new systems would be regulated to ensure safeguarding of patient care and safety through inspections by the Care Quality Commission.

Policy documents

Policy documents set out a vision for the future. They are not enshrined in law but they provide a common view of how health care could be, for example, costed or delivered. The most recent example of this for England is the aforementioned *Five Year Forward View* (Department of Health 2014), which attempted to provide a consensus on what future services could look like and how they could be delivered. The *Five Year Forward View* document recognises that a 'one size fits all' model of health care delivery does not work for every region and that new approaches, co-designed with the public, are required to meet the needs of local communities. This has resulted in the development of 'vanguard sites'.

In March 2015, the first 29 vanguard sites were chosen and they represented three different types: integrated primary and acute care systems; enhanced health in care homes and multispecialty community provider vanguards with eight urgent and emergency vanguards announced in July; and a further 13 acute care collaborations in September. Each vanguard will take on a lead in the development of new care models and will act as the blueprint for the NHS moving forward – *New Care Models* (Department of Health 2016).

This involves a root and branch redesign of whole health and care systems; and examples of suggestions from patients and service user groups have included: reducing numbers of trips to hospitals by having cancer and dementia specialists hold clinics in local surgeries; having one point of call for family doctors, community nurses, social and mental health services or access to blood tests; and having dialysis and chemotherapy services closer to home. Another aspect identified by patient groups as an area for improvement is reducing the confusing array of emergency and/or acute services for patients such as accident and emergency, GP out of hours, minor injury clinics, etc., so that patients can be seen by the right service at the right time in the right place.

Who regulates health and social care?

The Health and Safety Executive (HSE) is the national independent regulator for health and safety in the workplace. This includes private and publicly owned health and social care settings in Great Britain (and Northern Ireland). The HSE works in partnership with co-regulators in local authorities to inspect, investigate and, where necessary, take enforcement action. However, there are many other bodies in the devolved regions of the UK responsible for regulating health and social care and these are outlined below.

England

In England, the HSE has entrusted the Care Quality Commission (CQC) with the responsibility of dealing with most patient and service user serious health and safety incidents. The CQC is the lead inspection and enforcement body under the Health and Social Care Act 2008 for safety and quality of treatment and care matters involving patients and service users who are receiving a health or social care service from a provider registered with the CQC. It is an independent regulator whose purpose is to ensure that the health and social care sectors provide people with safe, effective, compassionate and high-quality care in England. They do this by maintaining a register of care providers, monitoring and inspecting services to ensure that they meet fundamental standards, and publishing their findings, including inspection ratings from 'outstanding' to 'inadequate'. Inspections can either be planned or unplanned. However, Sir Robert Francis was critical of both the CQC and regulatory bodies such as the General Medical Council (GMC) and the Nursing and Midwifery Council (NMC) in his report on the Mid Staffordshire NHS Foundation Trust (Francis 2013) in view of their lack of timely action and lack of response to patient complaints and staff concerns.

It is highly likely that, at some point in your professional career, the area you work in will be inspected by the CQC. There are five key questions that the CQC ask of all services they inspect:

- Are they safe? (In other words, are service users protected from abuse and avoidable harm?)
- Are they effective? (Is the care that service users receive underpinned by the best evidence?)
- Are they caring? (Do staff treat service users with compassion, dignity, kindness and respect?)
- Are they responsive to people's needs? (Are services organised to meet service users' requirements?)

- Are they well led? (Does the leadership, management and governance of the organisation ensure that it provides high-quality care based on individual need, encourages learning and innovation, and promotes an open and fair culture?)

From 1 April 2016, 'Monitor' was absorbed into the NHS as another mechanism to address quality. Monitor (NHS) is an executive non-departmental public body sponsored by the Department of Health initially to oversee the financial viability of Foundation Trusts and subsequently all NHS Trusts, as well as independent providers that provide NHS-funded care. Monitor (NHS) is the regulator for health services in England and has four core responsibilities:

- making sure public providers are well led and delivering quality care on a sustainable basis
- making sure essential NHS services are maintained
- making sure the NHS system promotes quality and efficiency
- making sure procurement, choice and competition operate in the best interests of patients.

Monitor works closely with the CQC to support improvements in the quality of care delivered by providers of NHS services and to promote the provision of well-led and sustainable services for the benefit of people who use health services.

Wales

The Healthcare Inspectorate Wales (HIW) (Welsh Government 2016a) is the independent inspectorate and regulator of all health care in Wales. The role of HIW is to review and inspect NHS and independent health care organisations. Services are reviewed against a plethora of published standards, policies and guidance. Furthermore through the inspection process, HIW provides assurance for patients, the public, Welsh government and health care providers in terms of quality, safety and effectiveness of services and will make recommendations to promote improvements.

The Care and Social Services Inspectorate Wales CSSIW (Welsh Government, 2016b) regulates social care, early year services and Local Authority care support services. This includes the registration of social care professionals, inspection of services, responding to concerns raised about regulated services, compliance support and enforcement.

Northern Ireland

The Regulation and Quality Improvement Authority (RQIA) is Northern Ireland's independent health and social care regulator and performs this duty through a programme of inspections and reviews. The RQIA monitors the availability and quality of health and social care services to ensure that they are accessible, well managed and meet the required standards. They aim to ensure that there is openness, clarity and accountability in the management and delivery of these services. The RQIA was established under the Health and Personal Social Services (Quality, Improvement and Regulation) (Northern Ireland) Order 2003. This Order is part of the devolved power for Ireland and the Department of Health (one of nine Northern Ireland Departments) which sets standards by which the RQIA inspects.

The RQIA has a Memorandum of Understanding (MoU) with the Health Care and Professions Council (HCPC) and has established a framework to support the working relationship between the RQIA and the HCPC in order to protect the wellbeing of the public receiving health and social care in Northern Ireland. Therefore any breaches of standards of care by an HCPC-regulated professional will be reported to the registration department of the HCPC and this may lead to disciplinary action, including warnings, suspension and ultimately dismissal.

Scotland

In April 2011, the Social Care and Social Work Improvement Scotland (SCSWIS) was created to scrutinise social care, social work and child protection services. In September 2011, they were renamed the Care Inspectorate. The Care Inspectorate regulates and inspects care services in Scotland. It has a number of strategic objectives (Care Inspectorate 2015), including those listed below. It aims:

- to provide assurance and build confidence through robust regulation and inspection
- to contribute to building a rights-based, world-class care system in Scotland
- to support people to understand the meaning of high-quality, safe and compassionate care by promoting the standards and quality of service they should expect and making sure their voices are heard
- to build capacity within care services to make sure there is high-quality development and improve 'rights-based care' across Scotland.
- to support and inform local and national policy development by providing high-quality, evidence-based advice and information
- to perform effectively and efficiently as an independent body and work in partnership with others.

Healthcare Improvement Scotland

Healthcare Improvement Scotland (HIS) was formed on 1 April 2011. The scope of HIS is to reduce health-associated infection risk to hospital patients, to improve the care of older adult patients, and to regulate independent health services through an inspection framework. Not unlike the Care Quality Commission, this is achieved by inspectors carrying out announced and unannounced inspections in acute NHS hospitals in Scotland to check that the NHS Quality Improvement Standards (QIS) standards for older people in acute care and standards for prevention and control of healthcare-associated infection are being met. It is also part of the national health care improvement organisation for Scotland and part of NHS Scotland. It consists of a number of organisations (Scottish Medicines Consortium, Scottish Health Technologies, Health Improvement Inspectorate; Scottish Patient Safety, Health Environment Inspectorate and Scottish Intercollegiate Guidelines Network).

Their work programme supports the health care priorities of the Scottish Government and they inspect care in hospitals, GP practices and NHS boards, and work with members of the public and professionals to improve the quality of health care. Their objectives are (Healthcare Improvement Scotland 2016):

- supporting and empowering people to have an informed voice in managing their own care and shaping how services are designed and delivered
- delivering 'scrutiny activity', which is fair but challenging and leads to improvements for patients
- providing quality improvement support to health providers
- providing clinical standards, guidelines and advice, based on the best available evidence.

Implications for health care practitioners

From a practitioner's perspective, there are independent inspectorates in each country, with health and social care coming under the auspices of one inspectorate in England and Northern Ireland, while in Wales and Scotland there are two separate inspectorates: one for health and one for social care. All health and social care practitioners should be familiar with their own country's inspectorate procedures and ensure they comply with them.

However, the existence of regulatory bodies and inspections still does not prevent tragedies from happening. Following the death of Baby P in 2008, the Secretary of State for Children, Schools and Families commissioned Lord Laming (who had previously chaired the inquiry into the death of Victoria Climbié in 2000 and published reports in 2003 and 2009) to undertake a review of the failings that led to Baby P's death. The first Laming Report, in 2003, considered a number of non-accidental deaths in children and identified some common themes:

- failure of communication between different staff and agencies
- inexperience and lack of skill of individual social workers

- failure to follow established procedures
- inadequate resources to meet demands.

The Health Select Committee reviewed and agreed with many of Lord Laming's key recommendations, chief of which was the proposed introduction of a new National Agency for Children and Families to ensure that police, health and housing services could carry out their duties effectively and efficiently. Furthermore, this agency would scrutinise new laws, ensure policy is implemented and could carry out serious case reviews. The introduction of these recommendations should prevent this type of tragedy from happening again. However, as we know to our cost, this is not always the case.

In 2009, with the death of 'Baby P', it became clear that many of the recommendations had not been put in place. Despite this, Lord Laming credited the government with the introduction of some new legislation and guidance to safeguard children. Some of the main features of safeguarding include identification, assessment, a focus on the child (as opposed to family, carer or relative in charge), analysis and outcomes and appropriate timeliness for action if needed. Nevertheless, there have been other tragedies which have highlighted significant failings in communication between different professionals and/or an unwillingness to speak out when poor practice is observed.

One change aimed at improving communication between professionals across different agencies was the introduction of interprofessional education. The origins of interprofessional education (IPE) lie in the work of Barr (1996) and the development of the Centre of Interprofessional Education (CAIPE). In the late 1980s, a number of groups/professionals from primary care, the community, learning disabilities, mental health and older adult care converged into a single movement, thus paving the way for the establishment of IPE nationwide from the late 1990s (Barr 1996). Since then, momentum has increased, particularly in the health and social care sector, since poor communication between different professionals and agencies has been implicated in the failings that resulted in the death of Victoria Climbié and Baby P.

Interprofessional education is now included in the HCPC *Standards of Proficiency* (2013), the HCPC *Standards of Conduct, Performance and Ethics* (2016) and the HCPC *Standards of Education and Training* (2017) as well as the NMC's *The Code: Professional Standards of Practice and Behaviour for Nurses and Midwives* (NMC 2015). Much emphasis has been placed on the need for universities to provide interprofessional education – in the hope that student professionals who learn together will work together more effectively in practice.

Reflective questions

- As a health or social care student (or new practitioner), reflect on your experiences of interprofessional learning.
- To what extent (if any), did these experiences improve communication between different professions?

Professional regulation

Health care professionals working within the NHS are regulated to make sure they have the skills needed to care for patients and that they treat everyone with respect and dignity. Depending on the particular profession, there are several regulatory bodies that monitor the professionalism and standards of conduct of health and social care professionals (see Chapter 1 for more details). The largest body for the regulation of allied health professionals is the HCPC, which currently regulates 16 professions:

- Art therapists
- Biomedical scientists
- Chiropodists/Podiatrists
- Clinical scientists
- Dieticians
- Hearing aid dispensers
- Occupational therapists
- Speech and language therapists
- Orthoptists
- Paramedics
- Physiotherapists
- Prosthetists
- Radiographers
- Practitioner psychologists
- Operating department practitioners
- Social workers (not in Wales).

The NMC is the regulatory body for all branches of nursing and midwifery and there is also the General Medical Council (GMC) for doctors. The HCPC, NMC and GMC are 'pan UK', which means that registrants are allowed to work in any of the four countries in Great Britain and Northern Ireland.

A regulatory body sets the training standards that a health care professional needs to attain for that role. It also keeps a register of qualified professionals and only those on the register are allowed to practise. Some bodies require their members to undertake courses and/or set aside an amount of time for continuing professional development (CPD) each year. The important thing, as a health care professional, is to ensure that you are familiar with the relevant regulatory body's policies and that you practise appropriately to your level of professional knowledge and skill. A proportion of the registered population is audited every two years to determine whether they have maintained their proficiency to practise. A regulatory body will investigate complaints made about a professional and, in serious cases, it can remove the professional's right to practise so that patients are protected from harm.

As well as regulatory bodies, individual professions also have professional associations that oversee practice, such as the Chartered Society of Physiotherapy. Please see Table 8.1 for a summary of the differences between regulatory and professional bodies. Regardless of these distinctions, all health and social care professionals should be familiar with the standards of conduct and behaviour required by *both* their regulatory body and their professional body.

Table 8.1 Differences between regulatory and association/professional bodies

Regulatory body	Association/Professional body
Acts in the interest of the public and has processes. Open and accountable to the public and the profession.	Acts in the interest of the profession.
Independent of professional bodies.	Independent of the regulatory body.
Promotes the process of regulation.	Promotes and supports the practitioners and the profession. Many professional bodies provide information on insurance for members.
Administers a single register of practitioners who meet agreed criteria.	A membership organisation of professional practitioners.
Works with the profession to agree and oversee minimum standards.	Ensures members meet its own standards which are at least those required by the regulatory body but may exceed them.
Sets requirements for generic continuing professional development (CPD).	Ensures members meet requirements for CPD.
Publishes code of conduct and/or ethics.	Has an ethical code for members, which would at least reflect the ethical code required by the regulatory body.

Has a council (or governing body) which includes both lay and professional representatives.	May also have a council or governing body with lay representation.
Has a published complaints and disciplinary procedure.	May also have a complaints and disciplinary procedure.
Liaises with government and other organisations when required.	If necessary, will liaise between practitioners and the regulatory body in the case of a complaint.
Enforces 'fitness to practise' procedures to remove practitioners from the register, if necessary.	Ensures that professional pre-registration programmes cover the core curriculum.

(Adapted from the General Regulatory Council for Complementary Therapies Factsheet, 2016)

Reflective questions
- Think about the regulatory standards for your profession and the ethical codes set out by your professional body.
- In what ways do these reflect the values and priorities identified in health and social care legislation within your area of the UK?

Conclusion

This chapter has focused on the political and legal interface with professional practice. It has considered the policy-making process and some key legal frameworks that are pertinent to current health and social care practitioners. Whilst the countries that make up the UK differ in terms of their health priorities and policies, there are some common principles which they all share. Firstly, they all need to provide effective and efficient services that reflect what matters to service users. In addition, they all focus on providing good-quality services and have developed mechanisms/inspectorates to monitor services, often in response to an example of pernicious practice (such as the case of 'Baby P'). As a health or social care professional, you need to be aware of the policies and law that govern your practice and take responsibility for ensuring that all your interventions are safe, respectful and person-focused. Above all, you need to ensure that your practice is within the scope of your professional knowledge and skills.

Reflective questions
- Reflect on the differences between legislation and policy in health and social care.
- Identify a local policy that directly impacts upon your professional practice and consider the legislative drivers that shape this policy.

References

Barr, H. (1996). Ends and Means in Interprofessional Education: Towards a Typology. *Education for Health*. **9**, 341–52.

Care Quality Commission (2016). *The Care Quality Commission: The Independent Regulator of Health and Social Care in England*. https://:www.cqc.org.uk/ (last accessed 16.12.2016).

The Care Inspectorate (2015). *The Care Inspectorate*. http://www.careinspectorate.com (last accessed 16.12.2016).

Department of Health (2010). *Equity and Excellence: Liberating the NHS*. London: The Stationery Office.

Department of Health (2013). *Health and Social Care Act*. London: The Stationery Office.

Department of Health (2014). *Five Year Forward View*. London: The Stationery Office.

Department of Health (2015). *The NHS Constitution for England*. London: The Stationery Office.

Department of Health (2016). *New Care Models: Vanguards – developing a blueprint for the future of NHS and Care Services*. London: The Stationery Office.

Francis, R. (2013). *Report of the Mid Staffordshire NHS Foundation Trust. Public Inquiry*. London: The Stationery Office.

General Regulatory Council for Complementary Therapies (2016). *Regular or Association?* http://www.grcct.org/regulation/regulator-or-association (last accessed 15.12.2016).

Gov.UK (2016). *Monitor*. https://www.gov.uk/government/organisations/monitor (last accessed 16.12.2016).

Health Care and Professions Council (2017). *Standards of Education and Training*. http://www.hcpc-uk.co.uk/assets/documents/10000BCF46345Educ-Train-SOPA5_v2.pdf (last accessed 05.07.2017).

Health Care and Professions Council (2016). *Standards of Conduct, Performance and Ethics*. http://www.hcpc-uk.co.uk/assets/documents/10004EDFStandardsofconduct,performanceandethics.pdf (last accessed 01.09.2017).

Health and Care Professions Council (2013). *Standards of Proficiency*. http://www.hpc-uk.org/aboutregistration/standards/standardsofproficiency (last accessed 16.12.2016).

Healthcare Improvement Scotland, (2016). *Healthcare Improvement Scotland: Official Site*. http://www.healthcareimprovementscotland.org (last accessed 16.12.2016).

Kennedy, I. (2010). *Learning from Bristol: The Report of the Public Inquiry into Children's Heart Surgery at the Bristol Royal Infirmary 1984–1995*. London: The Stationery Office.

Laming, H. (2003). *The Victoria Climbié Inquiry*. London: The Stationery Office.

Laming, H. (2009). *The Protection of Children in England: A Progress Report*. London: The Stationery Office.

NHS Public Health Wales (2012) *1000 Lives Plus*. http://www.1000livesplus.wales.nhs.uk/hcai (last accessed 26.09.2017)

NHS Scotland (2016). *National Musculoskeletal Advice and Triage Service MATS*. http://www.knowledge.scot.nhs.uk/msk/msk-national-advice-and-triage-service.aspx (last accessed 30.9.2017).

Nursing and Midwifery Council (2015). *The Code, Professional Standards of Practice and Behaviour for Nurses and Midwives*. https://www.nmc.org.uk/standards/code. (last accessed 16.12.2016).

Welsh Government (2016a). *The Healthcare Inspectorate Wales*. http://hiw.org.uk/ (last accessed 1.9.2017).

Welsh Government (2016b). *Care and Social Services Inspectorate Wales*. https://www.cssiw.org.uk (last accessed 1.9.2017).

Chapter 9

Duty of quality in times of constraint

Sally Abey and Matt Cole

Learning outcomes
By the end of this chapter you will be able to:
- Explain how market forces impact on health and social care
- Describe how health services are commissioned in the United Kingdom
- Reflect on how a new practitioner can be an investment and a resource
- Find evidence to support theories on how quality and efficiency in health and social care can be protected and maintained
- Describe the value of being an educator for future practitioners
- Demonstrate an awareness of entrepreneurship in public sector settings.

Introduction
At a time of austerity and constraint, maintaining quality within the health or social care setting can be challenging, as resources become tighter and more scrupulously controlled. This reduction in resources is taking place against a backdrop of inflationary pressures and increasing demand for services that are more responsive, resilient and efficient year on year. This is no longer solely the concern of managers, but is also the very real responsibility of all staff, clinical and non-clinical, graduate and student.

Emerging models of service provision and commissioning, combined with governance drives on quality and efficiency, are pushing boundaries and challenging 'old ideas'. The educational experience of future practitioners as undergraduates must encompass these principles, along with resilience and a readiness to expect change and take part in innovative problem solving. Economic and governance issues are changing the way health and social care professionals work and think. A whole new world of inclusive responsibility and accountability (beyond hands-on clinical care) is emerging and this is a challenge for new and experienced professionals alike.

As described throughout this chapter, England has undergone major reforms to the structure of the NHS, whilst Scotland and Wales have followed a more traditional model, with their governments retaining significant control over their health care. Northern Ireland's structure differs, again. The health and social care sector there works in an integrated way to provide health services. (See Chapter 6 for further discussion of the different organisational arrangements in the devolved nations of the UK.)

Health and social care as a marketplace

The idea of health and social care as a marketplace is a long way from Aneurin Bevan's initial vision of the NHS, based on the idea that providing free health care would make it possible to reduce sickness and disability, leading to improved levels of public health at all levels of society. Unfortunately, the reality of delivering that vision has proved very costly and the financial investment now runs into billions of pounds of public expenditure each year. This huge cost is partly due to medical advances – though rising public expectations (Appleby 2013), increased life-expectancy and a growing population also play their part. The burden of delivering high-quality and effective services, whilst ensuring that all areas are cost-efficient, is challenging. Cost and wastage are major problems. For instance, within the area of pharmaceuticals, an estimated £300 million is lost annually to prescribed drugs which are not used (Hazell & Robson 2015).

The NHS is a highly complex organisation encompassing a huge variety of professions delivering specialist aspects of medical care (Kinder & Burgoyne 2013). With an anticipated rise in complex chronic long-term health issues in an ageing population (Behan et al. 2013), the cost of running the NHS is set to continue rising, However, this financial burden is considered unsustainable and successive governments have sought ways to reduce costs whilst improving efficiency and quality. This has led to public policy that strives for more integrated working between 'care' providers resulting in the Health and Social Care Act (2012) (Department of Health 2015). The joining of health and social care heralds a change to established working practices across NHS and social care settings, presenting opportunities for more integrated working between a variety of health and social care professions in the delivery of patient-centred care.

The aim is to increase the quality of care, with improved outcomes delivered in a more cost-effective way. To achieve this, innovative ways of working are needed to make the required transformations (Priest 2012), in a climate of financial constraint. Consequently, the health care system's character has changed, with the formation of a marketplace promoting efficiency, cost-effectiveness and choice. A critical part of that process has been to establish local commissioning of services through clinical commissioning groups (CCGs) in NHS England, planning of patient pathways and, importantly, quality assurance.

However, whilst independent NHS contactors (such as general practitioners) deliver the majority of primary medical care across the NHS, the public perception of competition and the 'internal market' is perhaps of creeping privatisation. Independent contractors are not new to the NHS, but the concept of private companies providing services is a relatively new phenomenon that has evolved from the division between commissioners and providers of services, which started in the 1990s.

The use of competition varies across the four nations of the UK, with Scotland and Wales removing their internal markets in 2004 and 2009 respectively. Northern Ireland continues to utilise elements of competition, but the largest number of changes have been seen in NHS England. This variation is mostly due to the differing political stance of the relative devolved powers and their differences in scale, culture and history (Bevan et al. 2004).

The role of clinical commissioning groups in NHS England

The commissioning driver encourages health care provision to meet the need of the socio-demographic area it is serving, rather than taking a 'one size fits all' approach. However, this strategy also presents challenges, as it relies on the commissioners' ability to understand the needs of that community and its service users.

Social enterprise was originally viewed as an opportunity for service providers to create not-for-profit organisations providing services that could be delivered competitively, thereby minimising costs and winning contracts from other competitors. This interpretation is misleading, however, as a profit is essential in order to maintain an organisation's financial viability. Any profit is put back into the services provided to improve patient care, or benefit the community, whilst enabling the organisation to manage salaries and other inflation-related costs (Addicott 2011). Another initiative designed to increase patient choice across a number of services was 'any qualified provider' (AQP) to deliver health care services for the NHS in England. Essentially the 'provider' tenders to deliver services and must be able to demonstrate they can meet the qualification criteria set and overseen by the Care Quality Commission (CQC), NHS Improvement and the NHS Commission Board who, between them, check quality, cost and efficacy of provision (Speed & Gabe 2013).

How does commissioning work?

Commissioning works in the following way: the general practitioner makes a patient referral to a specialist service, and the patient is presented with a list of providers from which to choose. The service provider may already be established in the NHS, or come from a range of sources such as a charity or social enterprise or from the independent sector. However, since 2013 there has been no requirement for commissioners to use AQP; and in 2013/14 only 77 of the 183 CCGs sought other providers of open services to increase choice and competition via AQP (The King's Fund 2015).

Commissioning challenges

The concept of 'private' providers within the NHS has historically been a cause of contention amongst both politicians and the public (Collier & Scally 2015, The King's Fund 2015). These long-standing debates have been made more complex and intense by the drive to reduce the cost burden of the NHS for all four constituent UK nations, regardless of their stance on competition, efficiency and effectiveness. Whilst such factors rightly deserve constant scrutiny, the NHS in the UK continues to provide the best quality care and the most accessible and efficient service, compared to those of other nations worldwide (Davis *et al.* 2014). The advantage of commissioning private providers is that it creates competitiveness around cost efficiency and patient choice. However, as the example of the United States demonstrates, this model also has significant social and economic drawbacks, such as patients failing to gain access to health care due to costs being prohibitive (Davis *et al.* 2014).

Influences within the marketplace

In the wake of the Francis Report (Francis 2013) and subsequent cultural changes within the NHS, a patient-centred approach has been strongly established, engaging patients through such means as the 'Friends and Family Test' and patient surveys. This allows service users to provide feedback which influences decision-making and future service planning. Alongside these initiatives has been the introduction of the legal duty of candour in England, under the Health and Social Care Act (2008) whereby mistakes, however large or small, are communicated to the individuals involved and apologies made, whether or not the patient is aware of an issue.

Reporting of patient safety incidents has also become central to the clinical culture, with 'near misses' and 'never events' communicated through the management tiers to the Chief Executive and National Patient Safety Agency. Central to clinicians' practice is the provision of information to assist patients in making informed decisions regarding their own care. This has extended to patient and public involvement (PPI) regarding how health and social care services are provided (Mockford *et al.* 2012). The service user has a voice and agency to drive change regarding care delivery. As the recipient of care services, it is recognised that patients are well placed to provide insight and relevant commentary relating to their experiences.

New practitioners as an investment and resource

Strategies for promoting productivity and utilising resources focus on interprofessional learning and working. However, such an approach has the potential to create a 'market force', placing pressure on professional boundaries. There are also regulations and controls, such as professional scope of practice, which will influence how this is implemented (Nancarrow & Borthwick 2005). Working collaboratively towards shared goals, whilst offering profession-specific expertise, is the essence of interprofessional working (Hall 2005). To embed working across clinical settings by health professionals and to meet the needs of the patient, future leaders within health care need to be focused on the patient. This requires them to behave in such a way as to foster an environment where change thrives, but where the patient's own needs are uppermost (NHS England 2014). A report by NHS England, *Building and Strengthening Leadership*, challenges individual practitioners, teams, managers and organisations to take collective responsibility for the patient's welfare through compassionate leadership. To this end, clinicians are expected to embody attitudes and behaviours such as self-awareness, resilience, mindfulness and emotional intelligence (NHS England 2014), as well as clinical skills across the range of bandings and roles within each profession.

Undoubtedly, the roles of health care professionals are changing, with interprofessional working, leadership and change management becoming essential requirements, and this is reflected in the undergraduate training of students (Kinnair *et al.* 2012, McMurtry 2010, Scarvell & Stone 2010). It is incumbent upon higher education institutions (HEIs) to ensure that health care students are exposed throughout their training to other related professions, with opportunities to gain insight into their capabilities and be respectful of their skills and expertise (see also Chapter 7). Crucially, professionals need to graduate feeling confident about their own professional boundaries, competent to undertake their duties and open to new ways of working alongside other professions.

Reflective questions

- How confident are you, in terms of your own professional identity?
- What skills and knowledge differentiate you from other professionals with whom you work?
- To what extent did your undergraduate training equip you with qualities needed for practice, such as self-awareness and resilience?

Value of the clinical educator's role

The nomenclature used to define the role of 'clinical educator' varies in its meaning across professions, but the term 'clinical educator' will be used here to encompass 'mentor', 'practice educator', 'clinical teacher', 'preceptor', 'practice education facilitator' and 'clinical supervisor', representing an experienced professional working with students to develop their clinical skills. The clinical educator has a key role in the development of learners in terms of skills, practice, professionalism and confidence building.

Health care delivery continues to change and evolve, and individual professions must adapt and develop, with clinical educators not only being custodians but also visionaries with the power to inspire and influence the scope and ambitions of the next generation of professionals. The value of the clinical educator's role should not be underestimated and the personal challenge of undertaking this role, if appropriately managed and supported, can be extremely rewarding. Practice placement learning provides real-world experience within a complex and dynamic clinical setting (Bellman *et al.* 2003), where clinical educators are able to manage and help students interpret spontaneous interactions. Clinical educators also play an important part in the education of health care students by acting as role models through their own evidence-based practice, and their personal and professional behaviours. As facilitators and evaluators of student learning, clinical educators create an environment where student learning can flourish (Hinchliff 1992, Magginson & Clutterbuck 2005, Neary 2000, Rose & Best 2005).

Provision of high-quality, effective and efficient health care student placement learning is therefore critical for safeguarding staff and patients (Barker *et al.* 2011, O'Keefe *et al.* 2012). Clinical educators are an essential component of the workforce, providing health care for patients and mentorship for the next generation of health care professionals. Students are a subset of the health care workforce, working with service users under the supervision of clinical educators. The clinical educator is exceptionally well placed to influence the next generation of practitioners, establishing high standards of practice and introducing students to working interprofessionally.

Students bring with them a new perspective, which the clinical educator can harness and guide within this complex environment, encouraging creativity and innovation. HEIs have a role to play in inspiring this mindset, one example being Plymouth University's 'Enabling Practice Innovation Challenge'. This has helped develop new innovations in health, such as the smart catheter (iPee), which warns carers by text message if a patient's urine flow ceases, and a plaster cast that changes colour to indicate infection (Plymouth University 2016).

Reflective questions
- Reflect on your student clinical experience.
- Who were your best or favourite educators?
- What qualities did they possess?

Efficiency and good-quality health care

Educating new health care professionals creates challenges for efficiency and quality of health care, whilst shaping the responsibilities and roles of modern health professionals. There are multiple efficiency and quality drivers within the NHS, and these are motivated by many factors including targets for clinical expenditure, estates, procurement, governance, training and safeguarding of both service users and staff. With additional waiting time targets, large clinic lists and the unpredictable extra 'on the day' demands facing most services, supervision of students can be perceived as time-consuming and difficult for service managers and clinicians. Quality, efficiency and effectiveness are inextricably linked through NHS policy, and managing these three competing components is undeniably challenging. Placement learning does present a challenge with regard to maintaining quality and safety of care whilst providing the student with the required learning opportunities, offset against the potential impact on patient contacts.

Maintaining efficiency and quality in the practice learning environment

At a macro level, practice-based learning offers the student the opportunity to become acquainted with political landscapes, policy drivers, changes and provision of quality care whilst also maintaining efficiency and being effective. At a micro level, the student is exposed to the shared and individual agendas of the student/patient/clinical educator encounter. Before a patient meets the student, there should always be transparency with regard to the involvement of students in patient care. The student's aim is to learn and gain experience, working towards gaining 'sign-off' on their portfolio of learning outcomes as stipulated by the relevant professional regulator, HEI and Quality Assurance Agency (QAA), which demonstrate the student's competency. Treating patients as people, rather than caseloads to be managed in the pursuit of learning outcomes, is critical.

Embedding ideas of patient safety and choice, quality of care, effectiveness and efficiency through mutually agreed, clinically appropriate and patient-acceptable decisions are all critical in the modern NHS. However, balancing accountability and responsibility for the resources used in patient care is just as important as developing clinical skills. During placements, there are opportunities to educate students in how to deliver a service that values quality and efficiency equally. Evidence-based practice is closely aligned to considerations of economics, and the National Institute for Health and Care Excellence (NICE) publishes guidelines regarding savings and productivity. One such tool is *Estimating Return on Investment for Interventions and Strategies to Increase Physical Activity* (NICE 2014), developed for use by commissioners and policy makers to help them determine the 'return' on their investment, should they decide to commission those interventions.

Patient safety and quality of care are of primary importance to the supervising clinician, with the student's needs coming second. Again, staff who are well-trained clinical educators, as well as excellent clinicians, are required to provide a context and rationale for making choices in patient care and making the best use of resources. The patient is primarily concerned with their diagnosis and/or treatment, whilst the clinical educator is orchestrating the encounter, seeking to fulfil everyone's needs whilst delivering high-quality care within the parameters of a treatment plan that will lead to a desirable outcome.

Given the complexities and pressures involved in working in a busy practice setting, clinical educators and hosting organisations could easily view the presence of students as a potential risk to quality and efficiency, to patient safety and to staff wellbeing. It is therefore important to work closely with HEIs and commissioning bodies to address concerns as they arise, in order to mitigate potential threats to the learning environment.

Clinical staff are already at risk from stress, job dissatisfaction, burnout and work-life imbalance (Chang *et al.* 2005, Clouston 2014). Bearing all this in mind, it is essential to ensure that being given responsibility of student mentorship does not contribute to these pressures. Firstly, clinical educators must have sufficient capacity to undertake the role of clinical education and manage the presence of students whilst continuing to deliver patient care. They also need to have time to meet the student outside clinical hours, and should be given the opportunity to volunteer for the role rather than having a policy that all clinical staff must be clinical educators. In the field of podiatry, giving clinical educators responsibility for learning outcome sign-off, whilst having a previous or existing relationship with the HEI involved, has been found to increase clinical educator capacity (Abey *et al.* 2013, 2015). Enhancements such as these can have cost implications or may not be easily implemented. However, they can significantly affect, not only the student's experience, but also the clinical educator's capacity to cope with this additional role.

Meeting the challenge of efficiency and quality

Health professions are changing and developing, with nationally driven agendas produced by professional bodies and government. *Agenda for Change* (NHS Employers

2017) has introduced the possibility for non-qualified staff to undertake specific allied support roles typically at NHS bands two, three and four as support workers, assistants and assistant practitioners respectively. Health care assistants represent a third of the caring workforce and are viewed as critical to the development of the NHS and social care (Cavendish 2013). Self-interested professional protectionism is unlikely to be effective in avoiding change, given public expectations that cost-effective, high-quality and timely care will be delivered. Health and social care professionals are therefore tasked with navigating this changing landscape, and utilising opportunities to increase their scope of practice. One good example of this is independent prescribing for physiotherapists and podiatrists, which meets the needs of patients more effectively in a single consultation (Borthwick et al. 2010).

Sustainable, integrated health and social care needs a workforce that is flexible, progressive, capable of devising and delivering change and future-proofed as far as possible. A dynamic, forward-thinking drive by professional bodies and HEIs is required if health professions are to flourish, alongside high-quality learning environments within the NHS. The complexities of integrated health and social care, together with rapid medical advances, continue to challenge the placement learning model where patients with complex co-morbidities prevail.

Entrepreneurship in the public sector setting

On graduation, the new health care practitioner completes their studies, following immersion within 'real world' environments. This training provides a wealth of experience and insight into working practices, culture and dynamics in a variety of different locations within the NHS and, in some cases, the independent sector too. During placement, students get a 'fly on the wall' perspective – they are often welcomed as part of a team, sharing downtime and staff meetings with their 'colleagues'. Over a three- or four-month placement, the student witnesses the reality of working life and this provides them with scope for investigation and evaluation.

Action research offers a methodical approach to this process of investigation and evaluation, providing a framework that can be employed to support change not just at a local level, but also on a larger scale. Action research embraces professional, educational and organisational change (Bellman 2001) providing a real-world perspective (Willis 2007) within a community or structure (Williamson et al. 2012). Issues and problems can be identified and become the focus of change, which may involve individuals or a team working together. Each member of such a team, particularly an interprofessional team, brings an in-depth understanding of their own professional history and sociocultural context (Baum et al. 2006). This is vital to the sharing of information, creating new understanding and ultimately breaking out of entrenched ways of working and thinking, leading to implementation of positive change in the workplace (Waterman *et al.* 2007). Experiencing situations as a student does have limitations, as the student's interpretation is restricted by their stage of learning and their views may be based on an incomplete or superficial understanding of the 'supercomplex' environment they are seeking to decode (Lea & Callaghan 2012). Part of this 'supercomplexity' relates to the fact that clinicians are constantly bombarded with information relating to new evidence-based practices, protocols and government papers (Barnett 2000). Nevertheless, these experiences become a resource for the student. Exposure to different ways of managing universal challenges, lines of communication, cultural differences, innovation and entrepreneurship can all be reviewed and tailored for a new environment.

For dynamic, forward-thinking clinician-led services to be established, clinicians require vision to initiate and engage with change, and the ability to collaborate across a range of health and social care professions and providers. A time of austerity, with its demand to save both time and money without impacting quality, can in fact be an effective catalyst for innovation and entrepreneurship (Somekh & Zeichner 2009). For instance, income generation from car parking charges, provision of occupational health services and retail outlets within the hospital setting are now commonplace, but were innovative (and sometimes controversial) at their inception. There are also examples of patient-focused initiatives, such as the Robin Community Assessment Hub at Livewell South West, Plymouth, where services work in close partnership, supporting patients to stay at home to prevent inappropriate admission to hospital. Services on offer include ECGs, blood screening, bladder scanning, and functional and mobility assessment, combining the expertise of nurses, occupational therapists, physiotherapists and social care staff with that of general practitioners.

Conclusion

Given the continual changes within the health and social care sector, clinical educators need to develop students' critical thinking abilities (Archer 2010), assist their reflective practices and enable them to be patient-centred, decisive and compassionate. By the time they graduate, health and social care professionals will have gained a number of other skills, such as problem solving, critical thinking and communication skills, which are all essential in the modern health and social care arena. They also require flexibility, the ability to manage change whilst remaining resilient, and an understanding of the critical changes required to meet particular outcomes. This requires reflection, openness, a willingness to listen to all stakeholder views and the motivation to make changes. Clinical educators and HEIs must engender a spirit of innovation and entrepreneurship in students, as newly qualified health care professionals are critical to bringing a novel perspective to old problems.

Reflective questions

- What 'fresh perspectives' might you bring to working practices within your team or organisation?
- How might you improve the efficiency and effectiveness of your service?

References

Abey, S., Lea, S., Callaghan, L., Cotton, D. & Shaw, S. (2013). The development of a scale to assess practitioner capacity to engage in clinical education. *Journal of Further and Higher Education*. **39** (09), 1–18.

Abey, S., Lea, S., Callaghan, L., Cotton, D. & Shaw, S. (2015). Identifying factors which enhance capacity to engage in clinical education among podiatry practitioners: an action research project. *Journal of Foot and Ankle Research*. **8** (1), 66–74.

Addicott, R. (2011). *Social Enterprise in Health Care*. London: The King's Fund.

Appleby, J. (2013). *Spending on Health and Social Care over the Next 50 Years. Why Think Long Term?* London: The King's Fund.

Archer, J.C. (2010). State of the science in health professional education: effective feedback. *Medical Education*. **44** (1), 101–108.

Barker, M., Blacow, L., Cosgrove, S., Howorth, N., Jackson, G. & Mcmahon, J. (2011). Implementation of 'sign-off' mentorship: different perspectives. *British Journal of Nursing*. **20** (19), 1252–55.

Barnett, R. (2000). University knowledge in an age of supercomplexity. *Higher Education*. **40**, 409–22.

Baum, F., MacDougall, C. & Smith, D. (2006). Participatory action research. *Journal of Epidemiology and Community Health*. **60** (10), 854–57.

Behan, D., Perkins, A., Cumming, I., Patrick, Z., Bennett, D., Dillon, A., Melton, P., Nicholson, D., Flory, D. & Selbie, D. (2013). *The NHS Belongs to the People: A Call to Action*. https://www.england.nhs.uk/wp-content/uploads/2013/07/nhs-belongs.pdf (last accessed 05.06.2016).

Bellman, L. (2001). Courage, faith and chocolate cake: requisites for exploring professionalism in action. *Educational Action Research*. **9** (2), 225–42.

Bellman, L., Bywood, C. & Dale, S. (2003). Advancing working and learning through critical action research: creativity and constraints. *Nurse Education in Practice*. **3** (4), 186–94.

Bevan, G., Karanikolos, M., Exley, J., Nolte, E., Connollly, S. & Mays, N. (2004). *The Four Health Systems of the United Kingdom: How do they Compare?* http://www.nuffieldtrust.org.uk/sites/files/nuffield/publication/140411_four_countries_health_systems_summary_report.pdf (last accessed 5.6.2016).

Borthwick, A.M., Short, A.J., Nancarrow, S.A. & Boyce, R. (2010). Non- medical prescribing in Australasia and the UK: the case of podiatry. *Journal of Foot and Ankle Research*. **3** (1), 1.

Cavendish, C. (2013). *The Cavendish Review: An Independent Review into Healthcare Assistants and Support Workers in the NHS and Social Care Settings.* London: Department of Health.

Chang, E.M., Hancock, K.M., Johnson, A., Daly, J. & Jackson, D. (2005). Role stress in nurses: review of related factors and strategies for moving forward. *Nursing and Health Sciences*. **7** (1), 57–65.

Clouston, T.J. (2014). Whose occupational balance is it anyway? The challenge of neoliberal capitalism and work-life imbalance. *British Journal of Occupational Therapy*. **77** (10), 507–15.

Collier, S. & Scally, G. (2015). Can private providers be trusted to run NHS hospitals after Hinchingbrooke? *British Medical Journal.* **289** (11), 8–10.

Davis, K., Stremikis, K., Squires, D. & Schoen, C. (2014). *Mirror, Mirror on the Wall: How the Performance of the U.S. Health Care System Compares Internationally.* New York: The Commonwealth Fund.

Department of Health (2015). *2010 to 2015 Government Policy: Health and Social Care Integration.* London: The Stationery Office.

Francis, R. (2013). *Report of the Mid Staffordshire NHS Foundation Trust Public Inquiry.* http://webarchive.nationalarchives.gov.uk/20150407084003/http://www.midstaffspublicinquiry.com/ (last accessed 5.9.2017).

Hall, P. (2005). Interprofessional teamwork: professional cultures as barriers. *Journal of Interprofessional Care.* **19**, 188–96.

Hazell, B. & Robson, R. (2015). *Pharmaceutical Waste Reduction in the NHS.* https://www.england.nhs.uk/wp-content/uploads/2015/06/pharmaceutical-waste-reduction.pdf (last accessed 5.6.2016).

Hinchliff, S. (1992). *The Practitioner as Teacher.* Edinburgh: Bailliere and Tindall.

Kinder, T. & Burgoyne, T. (2013). Information processing and the challenges facing lean healthcare. *Financial Accountability and Management.* **29** (3), 271–90.

Kinnair, D.J., Anderson, E.S. & Thorpe, L.N. (2012). Development of interprofessional education in mental health practice: adapting the Leicester Model. *Journal of Interprofessional Care.* **26** (3), 189–97.

Lea, S.J. & Callaghan, L. (2012). 'Teaching in an age of "supercomplexity": Lecturer conceptions in context' in P. Trowler, M. Saunders & V. Bamber (eds). *Tribes and Territories in the 21st Century.* Abingdon: Routledge.

Magginson, D. & Clutterbuck, D. (2005). *Techniques for Coaching and Mentoring.* London: Elsevier Ltd.

McMurtry, A. (2010). Complexity, collective learning and the education of interprofessional health teams: insights from a university-level course. *Journal of Interprofessional Care.* **24** (3), 220–29.

Mockford, C., Staniszewska, S., Griffiths, F. & Herron-Marx, S. (2012). The impact of patient and public involvement on UK NHS health care: a systematic review. *International Journal for Quality in Health Care: Journal of the International Society for Quality in Health Care/ISQua.* **24** (1), 28–38.

Nancarrow, S.A. & Borthwick, A.M. (2005). Dynamic professional boundaries in the healthcare workforce. *Sociology of Health and Illness.* **27** (7), 897–919.

National Institute of Health and Clinical Excellence (NICE) (2014). *Estimating Return on Investment for interventions and strategies to increase physical activity: User Guide.* London. NICE. https://www.nice.org.uk/Media/Default/About/what-we-do/Into-practice/Return-on-Investment/NICE-return-on-investment-physical-activity-user-guide.pdf (last accessed 16.10.2016).

Neary, M. (2000). Supporting students' learning and professional development through the process of continuous assessment and mentorship. *Nurse Education Today.* **20**, 463–74.

NHS Employers (2017). http://www.nhsemployers.org/your-workforce/pay-and-reward/agenda-for-change/nhs-terms-and-conditions-of-service-handbook (last accessed 5.9.2017).

NHS England (2014). *Building and Strengthening Leadership.* https://www.england.nhs.uk/wp-content/uploads/2014/12/london-nursing-accessible.pdf (last accessed 05.06.2016).

O'Keefe, M. Burgess, T. McAllister, S. & Stupans, I. (2012). Twelve tips for supporting student learning in multidisciplinary clinical placements. *Medical Teacher.* **34** (11), 883–87.

Plymouth University (2016). *Enabling Practice Innovation Challenge (EPIC).* https://www.plymouth.ac.uk/schools/school-of-nursing-and-midwifery/epic (last accessed 01.06.2016).

Priest, J. (2012). *The Integration of Health and Social Care.* London: British Medical Association Health Policy and Economic Research Unit.

Rose, M. & Best, D. (2005). *Transforming Practice through Clinical Education, Professional Supervision and Mentoring.* Edinburgh: Churchill Livingstone.

Scarvell, J.M. & Stone, J. (2010). An interprofessional collaborative practice model for preparation of clinical educators. *Journal of Interprofessional Care.* **24** (4), 386–400.

Somekh, B. & Zeichner, K. (2009). Action research for educational reform: remodelling action research theories and practices in local contexts. *Educational Action Research.* **17** (1), 5–21.

Speed, E. & Gabe, J. (2013). The health and social care act for England 2012: the extension of 'new professionalism'. *Critical Social Policy.* **33** (3), 564–74.

The Health and Social Care Act. (2008). London: The Stationery Office.

The King's Fund (2015). Is the NHS Being Privatised? http://www.kingsfund.org.uk/projects/verdict/nhs-being-privatised (last accessed 05.-6.2016).

Waterman, H., Marshall, M., Noble, J., Davies, H., Walshe, K., Sheaff, R. & Elwyn, G. (2007). The role of action research in the investigation and diffusion of innovations in health care: the PRIDE project. *Qualitative Health Research.* **17** (3), 373–81.

Williamson, G., Bellman, L. & Webster, J. (2012). *Action Research in Nursing and Healthcare.* London: Sage Publications Ltd.

Willis, J.W. (2007). *Foundations of Qualitative Research: Interpretive and Critical Approaches.* London: Sage Publications Ltd.

Chapter 10

Research in health and social care practice

Steven W. Whitcombe

Learning outcomes

By the end of this chapter you will be able to:
- Define research as a concept and discuss its value to health and social care practice
- Explicate key research paradigms and methodologies that frame research inquiry
- List ways of becoming 'research active' in the workplace
- Contemplate the potential of research as a career.

It is well recognised that practitioners in health and social care need to be consumers of research, to make sense of research findings, to evidence their practice and to justify their choice of interventions (Parahoo 2014). Moreover, the requirement to utilise research is embodied within the standards for professionals working in the care sector. For example, the Health and Care Professions Council's *Standards of Proficiency for Physiotherapists* (2013, 14.10) state that physiotherapists should 'be able to use research reasoning and problem-solving skills to determine appropriate actions'. Likewise, the Nursing and Midwifery Council's *The Code: Professional Standards of Practice and Behaviour for Nurses and Midwives* (2015, 8.4) asserts that nurses and midwives need the skills and knowledge to 'evaluate the quality' of their work.

    Most, if not all, pre-registration programmes in health and social care require students to develop an understanding of research design, methods and processes and to appreciate why research is important to their practice. However, whilst students may learn to be critical consumers of research, their knowledge of how to engage in research and the opportunities to do this as a new practitioner may not be so well established.

This chapter will consider the transfer of research knowledge and skills to the practice context. It will begin with an overview of what is meant by research and a reminder of its importance in health and social care. This will be followed by an examination of the paradigms that influence the design of research projects. The chapter will then focus on how to participate in research, whether you are just starting out on your career or you are a more experienced professional.

What is research?

Research can be defined as an investigation into a topic, or a means to answer a question on a given issue. It is best viewed as a systematic process, a form of rigorous inquiry that incorporates transparent (and ethical) methods of data collection, analysis and interpretation (Bryman 2012). The contribution of research to health and social care is largely three-fold. First, research can uncover new understandings of concepts that are common to our practice – for example, the meanings people attribute to client-centredness or person-centred care. Second, research can identify new solutions to problems in health and social care or new ways of delivering practice. That said, Parahoo (2014) reminds us that research is not only valuable in terms of discovering new approaches to care but it can also provide sound evidence for practice founded on tradition or a seemingly 'commonsense' way of doing things. This then leads to a third purpose – research can be used to evaluate the effectiveness of an intervention and offer evidence for the use of a treatment.

Research and science

The term 'science' is Latin in origin and its meaning is associated with the pursuit of knowledge. In this respect, the concepts of science and research appear to be one and the same but this depends on how rigidly you define 'science'. The classical connotations of science, or the 'scientific method' most associated with disciplines such as physics, biology or chemistry, began to gain ground in the Middle Ages and particularly during the 'Enlightenment' from around the eighteenth century onwards (Jones 2003). This period was characterised by a rise in secular forms of knowledge as a means to make sense of the world, as opposed to commonly held religious explanations.

This notion of science is concerned with the search for 'truth' – the development of 'universal laws' to explain or predict action or, in the case of people, human behaviour (May 2011). However, this is potentially problematic when the intention of research is not to predict human behaviour but to enhance our understanding of how people describe and interpret their lives and surroundings. Research of this kind is often localised and culturally specific, with no attempt to formulate universal laws of explanation. This dichotomy in our understanding of research and science has led to the creation of two distinct paradigms which influence how research is implemented – positivism and interpretivism. These two paradigms are admittedly very different but they are often conceived in a polarised way, which exaggerates their differences. In practice, their differences are less significant.

A research paradigm can be used to describe a body of beliefs; it defines what can legitimately be studied and how this should be done. In essence, research paradigms are concerned with 'ontological' and 'epistemological' issues (Bryman 2012). Ontology refers to our beliefs about the nature of reality, whether or not you as a researcher believe that the social world is external to the individual and therefore can be investigated in a detached way. Epistemology on the other hand is concerned with 'how we know what we know' and the most appropriate methods with which to acquire knowledge about the world.

Positivism as a research paradigm.

Positivism adheres to an 'objective ontological position'. It is rooted in the natural sciences such as physics, chemistry and biology. Its guiding principle is that 'if something exists in nature, it has been caused by something else in nature' (Jones 2003, p.10). Therefore, positivism is concerned with 'cause and effect' and the role of the researcher is to examine the 'cause and effect' relationships between phenomena in an objective, neutral and value-free way. Those of a positivist persuasion argue that we can 'only know what we know by what we sense' – i.e. by what we can see, hear or touch. Consequently, from an epistemological standpoint, positivists are interested in gathering empirical 'facts' about the world, or 'truths' that can be generalised from a sample of participants to a wider population (Bryman 2012). To achieve this, positivist researchers tend to adopt research methods such as experimentation and observation, which they employ in a 'deductive' fashion. That is, they tend to start with a hypothesis (a testable statement about the relationship between two or more variables). When subjected to scrutiny or testing, the hypothesis may be upheld or rejected.

Interpretivism as a research paradigm

Historically, those interested in studying social phenomena took their lead from the natural sciences and adopted a positivist approach to research. In the late nineteenth and early twentieth centuries, some of the founding fathers of sociology (including Auguste Comte and Emile Durkheim) viewed positivism as a means to create a 'science of society', to examine how societies are patterned and organised and even as a way to predict people's behaviour (Jones 2003).

However, writing around the same time as Durkheim, sociologists such as Max Weber (1949) started to challenge the appropriateness of positivism as an approach to studying human action. Through his notion of *versehen*, Weber argued that people consciously chose their actions, and social science should therefore be concerned with exploring *why* they choose to behave in certain ways and what motivates them to do this. This requires a different approach from positivism, since it tries to understand rather than predict human behaviour. Silverman (1997) points out that objections to positivism by social researchers gained further ground during the mid-twentieth century. At this time, authors such as Herbert Blumer and Alfred Schutz argued that positivists' focus on logic leads them to overlook the importance of social construction.

Such critiques laid the foundation for an 'interpretivist research paradigm', with its emphasis on understanding, describing and interpreting human behaviour (Taylor & Francis 2013). Here, the ontological position is centred around the concepts of subjectivity and social constructivism. Interpretivists argue that people's interpretation of the world (their lived experience) is governed by their social and historical context and this accounts for there being 'multiple truths', rather than a single explanation of human action. Moreover, the role of the researcher is not to distance themselves from their research but to recognise and acknowledge how their own world view, social position, values and knowledge will influence their research. According to interpretivists, it is only through a reflexive consideration (self-examination) of the researcher's influence that a study can achieve credibility (Gough 2003).

Regarding epistemology, researchers influenced by an interpretivist paradigm often use methods of data collection such as interviews, focus groups and unstructured observation. They frequently use 'inductive' rather than 'deductive' methods of inquiry. Their research is often focused on a particular setting and their goal is to 'uncover meanings' about particular phenomena that may not be statistically generalisable to a wider population but may nonetheless be transferable to other contexts (Harding 2013).

Reflective questions

- Reflecting on what you have read so far, think about which research paradigm relates most closely to how you make sense of the world.
- How might your preference for a particular paradigm influence the type of research that you choose to undertake?

Paradigm purity, theory and practice

An appreciation of research paradigms is unquestionably helpful when trying to unravel what motivates researchers, or when trying to understand different approaches to research design. As we have seen, there are particular methods of data collection that are common to the positivist or interpretivist paradigm; there are also broader methods of inquiry stemming from these different research traditions. For example, the interpretivist paradigm has led to specific research methodologies/frameworks, such as phenomenology, grounded theory and narrative inquiry. Unfortunately, space won't allow us to explore all these research methods here but they are well documented in most research textbooks.

However, there is a need for caution when rigidly applying what Delamont and Atkinson describe as a 'paradigm mentality' (1995, p.193) to research practice. Loyalty to a particular position has in the past led to skirmishes within the research community. Positivists have been accused of adopting over-controlling, dogmatic approaches to research design, whilst interpretivists have been accused of presenting woolly, subjective accounts of human experience. Furthermore, a major problem for those entrenched in the orthodoxy of a research paradigm is that it can negate a creative and innovative approach to the investigation of an issue. As Delamont and Atkinson (1995, p.206) eloquently note, ' there may often be merit in using the rhetoric of paradigms or traditions as a retrospective logic or accounting device: summarising trends, emphases, continuities, and contrasts. What is dangerous and misleading on the other hand is to translate them into prescriptions'. The same can be said of such labels as 'qualitative' and 'quantitative' research. Although the former (through its reliance on words and verbal expression) is most associated with the interpretivist paradigm, and the latter (through its application of numbers/ statistics) is most associated with the positivist paradigm, in practice such crude distinctions are of limited value. For instance, consider the two scenarios below:

> Scenario 1: A researcher is interested in evaluating the effectiveness of a falls prevention programme with the aim of reducing hospital readmission rates for those susceptible to falls.
>
> Scenario 2: A researcher is interested in people's experiences of living with a diagnosis of multiple sclerosis and the effects of this on their family lives, work and friendships.

In the first scenario, the desire to assess the 'effectiveness' of a falls prevention programme would suggest that the researcher would utilise quantitative research methods. In the second scenario, an emphasis on understanding people's experiences of living with a condition could lead to the use of qualitative methods. However, in this second scenario the researcher could equally adopt methods that are both qualitative (e.g. interviews) and quantitative (e.g. structured questionnaires), if the intention is to obtain data that has both breadth and depth. In practice such 'mixed methods' designs, which take a more holistic perspective, are becoming increasingly common. Correspondingly, when making pragmatic decisions about research design and which methods to use, the starting point must always be the research question itself. A clear research question and/or study aim should pave the way for the most appropriate research strategy.

Using research skills in practice

So far, this chapter has reviewed our understanding of research and the paradigms that frame research inquiry. The remainder of the chapter will concentrate on some suggestions for how to utilise and develop your own research skills and knowledge in the health and social care environment. The starting point for this could be the sharing of findings from your undergraduate/pre-registration research project. Many students in health and social care have to complete an empirical study (dissertation) as part of their degree, and the outcomes of these are seldom disseminated. Nevertheless, the dissemination of research results is an important part of the research process, however large or small the study. You don't have to necessarily publish your pre-registration research, or present at a conference. Simply discussing your work with your colleagues and engaging in this process sets you on the path of being 'research-active'. On this path, you will find that there are broadly two routes that you can take to remain engaged in research. The first of these requires you to develop links and make time to be involved in research within your work environment. The second route involves developing links with research-active communities outside your organisation.

Research collaboration in the workplace

To be a successful researcher and develop research skills and knowledge, you will have to communicate with others and find time for research in your daily work. As someone who is new to an organisation or as a relatively new practitioner, this may seem daunting and the least of your priorities as you try to get to grips with settling into a health or social care environment. You may be more concerned with honing your nursing/therapeutic skills, rather than dealing with research. However, you do have a professional responsibility to at least read and use research to evidence and justify your interventions. One way of achieving this is through being part of (or setting up) a monthly journal club or research forum where you and your colleagues can discuss articles of interest that are pertinent to your practice.

Also, as a new practitioner, you should take the opportunity to agree a set time (e.g. one day per month) with your line manager/mentor that will be dedicated to your engagement in research. This is not as unrealistic as it may sound and your employment contract may give you leverage to bargain for it. For example, if you are employed in the NHS, you will be working under *Agenda for Change* and the *NHS Knowledge and Skills Framework* (Department of Health 2004). This framework provides a means to develop the skills and knowledge of NHS employees throughout their careers as well as promoting the development of effective services.

If you work for a statutory health setting within the NHS or social care, find out who in that organisation has an active role in research and make contact with them. If you work for a Trust, your first port of call might be your research and development team. These are colleagues and they will be able to tell you about the research priorities of your workplace and how you can get involved.

Researching with others outside your organisation

One way of developing your research skills or participating in research projects is by developing links with your local universities. As Bernstein (2000) argues, universities are sites for knowledge production as well as reproduction. Consequently, most academic staff are expected to be research-active. You can find out about the research priorities of different universities through their mission/vision statements and more specifically their interests in health and social care research through their Faculty/School websites. Universities fund research through private investors or through grants awarded by research councils, such as the Medical Research Council or the Economic and Social Research Council. Through the Higher Education and Research Bill (House of Commons 2016), the government is currently proposing to abolish separate research councils in favour of one body ('United Kingdom Research and Innovation') as a means to streamline research funding in the areas of science, technology, humanities and new ideas.

Whilst health care academics may have particular research expertise, they will be keen for practitioners to be involved with their projects – especially since practitioners are situated at the clinical/research interface. Through developing links with the university sector, you may be able to gather data for studies in your area of practice, become part of a bigger team that develops or writes research proposals and learn how to apply for research grants. As a novice researcher, you can also apply for research funding from charities or professional bodies. For example, the Royal College of Occupational Therapists frequently offers grants as a means of expanding the evidence base for occupational therapy.

In the spirit of collaboration, there are also numerous research social networks that you can access via the Internet in order to make connections with others who are researching in your field. Lastly, if you want to grow your research skills and knowledge, you could think about postgraduate or higher degree study. In order to advance your career in health and social care, it is likely that you will have to undertake further qualifications such as a master's degree. Most master's programmes will include a research element but you could be more focused than this and opt for a specific research degree. There are various options, depending on whether you want to be a 'career researcher' or a 'researching professional'. If you want a career in research (usually in the university sector), you need to think about a master's/doctor of philosophy (PhD).

These can be studied part time (around five years) or full time (around three years) and you will need to carry out an extensive and original investigation into a particular issue, culminating in a thesis of around 60,000 to 100,000 words. As well as gaining expert knowledge of a particular topic, completing a PhD will also enable you to gain expertise in a particular research method or methods.

If, on the other hand, you wish to develop your research skills and remain in practice, you could undertake a professional doctorate. This type of qualification meets the same standard and rigour as the PhD but, as Brown (2006) points out, the key distinction lies in its focus. Professional doctorates are usually undertaken on a part-time basis and concentrate on research topics that are relevant to the practice context. This means that they are focused on work-based issues. Professional doctorates, such as those in health and social work, require candidates to undertake modular assignments or work-based portfolios, as well as a thesis of around 40,000 to 60,000 words. This type of doctorate is becoming a popular option for managers and/or future leaders of professions who have responsibility for embedding a research culture in the workplace. Some universities may offer specialised master's degrees (such as a Master's in Clinical Research), which are also aimed at practising professionals from health care settings. As well as providing a master's level award that can be used to apply research skills within the practice setting, these types of programmes are often a staging post leading towards a doctoral programme.

Conclusion

This chapter began with an overview of research and its importance in health and social care. Practitioners in health and social care have a professional responsibility to engage with research, both to evidence their interventions and to develop their knowledge and skills. This chapter has also identified various types of research with different intentions stemming from different paradigmatic traditions. However, it has been argued that 'the practice of research' is less polarised than the theoretical traditions from which research methods are derived. Ultimately it is the research question itself that will govern the most appropriate method/s of inquiry.

Finally, we have considered the transition of taught research skills into practice and offered some suggestions whereby the new (and more established) practitioner can become both a consumer and an agent of research. Although research is vital to the advancement of health and social care, it may seem laborious, dry or time-consuming. However, it need not be any of these. Research is challenging but it also provides a vehicle for a creative, pioneering approach to problem-solving and for discovering new insights into our practice and the world around us.

Reflective questions

- Think about your own area of practice. How could research help to evidence your interventions?
- How could you become research-active in your own workplace?
- Who could help you engage with research and develop your research knowledge and skills?

References

Bernstein, B. (2000). *Pedagogy, Symbolic Control and Identity: Theory, Research, Critique.* (revised edn). Oxford: Rowman and Littlefield.

Brown, A. (2006). 'Language of Description and the Education of Researchers' in R. More, M. Arnot, J. Beck & H. Daniels (eds). *Knowledge, Power and Educational Reform, Applying the Sociology of Basil Bernstein.* London: Routledge.

Bryman, A. (2012). *Social Research Methods.* 4th edn. Oxford: Oxford University Press.

Delamont, S. & Atkinson, P. (1995). *Fighting Familiarity, Essays on Education and Ethnography.* Cresskill, New Jersey: Hampton Press.

Department of Health (2004). *The NHS Knowledge and Skills Framework (NHS KSF) and the Development Review Process.* London: Department of Health.

Gough, B. (2003). 'Deconstructing Reflexivity' in L. Finlay & B. Gough (eds). *Reflexivity: a Practical Guide for Researchers in Health and Social Sciences.* Oxford: Blackwell.

Harding, J. (2013). *Qualitative Data Analysis from Start to Finish.* London: Sage.

Health and Care Professions Council (HCPC) (2013). *Standards of Proficiency for Physiotherapists.* London: HCPC.

House of Commons (2016). *Higher Education and Research Bill.* London: The Stationery Office Ltd.

Jones, P. (2003). *Introducing Social Theory.* Cambridge: Polity Press.

May, T. (2011). *Social Research: Issues, Methods and Process.* 4th edn. Buckingham: Open University Press, McGraw-Hill Education.

Nursing and Midwifery Council (NMC) (2015). *The Code: Professional Standards of Practice and Behaviour for Nurses and Midwives.* London: NMC.

Parahoo, K. (2014). *Nursing Research, Principles, Process and Issues.* 3rd edn. Basingstoke: Palgrave MacMillan.

Silverman, D. (1997). 'The Logics of Qualitative Research' in G. Miller & R. Dingwall (eds). *Context and Method in Qualitative Research.* London: Sage.

Taylor, B. & Francis, K. (2013). *Qualitative Research in Health Sciences: Methodologies, Methods and Processes.* London: Routledge.

Weber, M. (1949). *The Methodology of the Social Sciences.* New York: Free Press.

Section 4
Caring values, spirituality, resilience and the duty of care

Introduction
By Teena J. Clouston

In this final section of the book we look at some of the more emotive and personal aspects of your practice and developmental transitions. These chapters have been placed at the end of the book because they are perhaps the most personally challenging, in that they ask you to consider who you really are, in terms of your personal values and beliefs. Moreover, and crucially, they ask you to adapt or change these, if necessary, to meet the needs of others in your everyday working practice.

Chapters 11 and 12 consider some critical issues regarding *duty of care* – the moral or legal obligation to ensure the well-being of others. Exploring the protection of vulnerable adults and children respectively, these chapters enable you to consider how these legal and moral obligations influence your own practice. They also provide an in-depth, historical overview to explain *why* these professional and ethical standards originally emerged and why they are relevant to contemporary practice. Although this can make challenging reading, it is a necessary journey because it tasks *you* with considering how you can prevent further adverse events happening in the future. This is about understanding *why* we have to raise concerns and enabling us to see ourselves as agents of *action* and *change*, both of which are necessary to meet the professional standards and ethics that frame practice.

The final three chapters in this section (Chapters 13, 14 and 15) look, respectively, at the more intangible elements – caring values, spirituality and resilience. These frequently overlooked aspects of practice are essential components of *personhood* and therefore require you to understand and question your own values and beliefs, as an individual person and a professional in practice. It is vital to know your 'self' and have the ability to make caring for others a genuine priority. Of course, this is not easy in contemporary health and social care environments because caring for others and their spiritual needs, as well as caring for yourself, is frequently disregarded in the drive to meet performance targets. How then do you prepare for this pressure and challenge it? These three chapters tackle these issues from a range of interlinking perspectives.

In order to get the most from these chapters, we ask that you really engage with and reflect on the questions and practical exercises you will find in them. It is only through an honest and meaningful exploration of your own beliefs and values that the full benefit of these last few chapters will be experienced.

Chapter 11
Safeguarding vulnerable adults

Gareth Morgan

Learning outcomes
By the end of this chapter you will be able to:
- Describe the process of safeguarding for vulnerable adults, and the ethical and moral issues it raises in both practice settings and daily life
- Understand what policy makers, services and professional organisations have done to ensure the protection of vulnerable adults and why this can be challenging to maintain at micro, meso and macro levels
- Consider the relevance and implications of safeguarding of vulnerable adults for professionals in health and social care settings and for you as an individual practitioner
- Contextualise the historical issues that demonstrate why safeguarding for vulnerable adults is so important in contemporary health and social care practice, and consider how this influences your practice, to instigate change and maintain standards of care.

Introduction

Adult protection has less of a social policy history, and has had less publicity, than child protection – perhaps because society has been unaware that vulnerable adults, who by their very nature are unable to protect themselves from others, have needed protection. However, in recent years, the notion of adult protection has been given the belated respect it deserves, perhaps partly because the ageing population is growing (Richardson 2014). This awakening mirrors the manner in which child abuse, as a concept, emerged into the public domain through disclosures and subsequent exposure in the media (Baeza 2008).

A brief historical overview: why do vulnerable adults need protection?

The issue of why we need to protect an adult has its roots in the somewhat chequered history of caring for the vulnerable in our society. Essentially, the way in which vulnerable adults have been cared for has not always been characterised or informed by their needs; quite the opposite, in fact. For instance, in the Middle Ages treatment commonly ranged from purging, bleeding and cold baths to beatings (Bloch & Singh 1999). Fast-forward a few centuries to the long-stay NHS Ely hospital, an NHS facility for people with learning disabilities (then called mental handicap) in Cardiff in the 1960s, and things were only marginally better. Despite the passing of laws such as the Idiots Act (1888) and the Inquiry into the Care of the Feeble Minded (1904), people were being admitted with medical diagnoses of 'imbecile' and 'idiot', these very terms introducing them to those who cared for them in the hospital as 'vulnerable' (Community Care 2007). An official inquiry into alleged abuse at the hospital in 1969 revealed that it was isolated from the community and wider health care environment and, with little staff training, abuse of vulnerable patients had proliferated (Department of Health and Social Security (DHSS) 1969).

A nursing assistant raised allegations that led to an inquiry in 1967; and this is significant, in that this insider informing (or 'raising concerns' as it is now known) would be repeated in other institutionally based scandals in later years. Specifically cited was cruel treatment, verbal abuse, beatings, pilfering of clothing and other items from patients, indifference to complaints, lack of medical care and frequent use of medication to sedate residents (DHSS 1969). Ely exposed the vulnerability of patients and compelled policy changes, altering the way government viewed long-stay institutions. It led to the 1971 white paper *Better Services for the Mentally Handicapped* (Department of Health (DH) 1971) and introduced regular visiting and inspection of such services (Community Care 2007).

In more recent times, the notion of vulnerability in the cared-for adult population has resurfaced in relation to older people. The phrase 'granny battering' first appeared in 1975 in an article in *Modern Geriatrics* (Baker 1975). Thereafter, at a conference in 1988, the British Geriatric Society focused on the urgent need for a response to the problem (McCreadie 2008). It was revisited in the 1990s when the Social Service Inspectorate published *Confronting Elder Abuse* (Sutton 1992), accompanied, shortly afterwards, by some specific guidelines entitled *No longer afraid: the safeguard of older people in domestic settings* (DH & Tomlinson 1993).

Yet, in the twenty-first century, the incidence of abuse continues seemingly unabated, with 1 in 20 adult patients having experienced abuse in the UK (Griffith 2015).

Of patients' relatives interviewed by the external committee investigating care at Tawel Fan ward, Acute Mental Health Unit, Glan Clwyd Hospital in Wales, 89% had very serious concerns about the care offered (Donna Ockenden Ltd 2014). The Harold Shipman scandal provided one of the most infamous reminders of the need to protect vulnerable adults (DH 2002a). Another was the systemic failure in the ongoing care of vulnerable patients in Mid-Staffordshire that led to an extensive inquiry into Mid-Staffordshire NHS Foundation Trust (see Preface). These failings were so extensive that the government commissioned a report by Robert Francis QC, known as the Francis Report (2013) thereafter, which became synonymous with institutional neglect and failings.

This report documented the appalling suffering of many patients within a secretive, defensive service culture and highlighted many examples of systemic failure. Yet these events occurred in an NHS that is often accused of over-regulation. Indeed, the system was supposed to have checks and balances in place, and its personnel should have been striving to ensure that patients were treated with dignity, and suffered no harm (see Chapter 13). The massive 1,782 page report contained 290 recommendations, which had major ramifications for all levels of the health service across England and stressed the need for a whole-service, patient-centred focus. The detailed recommendations did not call for a reorganisation of the system, but for a re-emphasis on what is important, to ensure that such systemic neglect in the care of the vulnerable would never recur (Francis 2013).

The Francis Report has impacted on care across the entire health and social care sector and all the devolved nations of the UK. Nevertheless, other smaller-scale care scandals have since occurred. For example, staff members from the Hillcroft Care Home in Lancashire were convicted of tormenting and abusing older residents (BBC News 2014). Residents were pelted with beanbags, mocked and bullied and the tormentors assumed their crime would remain undetected due to the residents' confused condition. As a result of cases like this, the use of overt and covert CCTV is now an accepted method of protecting people who are considered to be at risk of abuse in health and social care settings. The Care Quality Commission (2015) provides a useful overview for readers who are interested in the topic.

At the same time, the UK had seen a rise in policy that placed 'an increasing emphasis on the quality of health service provision' (Miller 2008, p.250). This rise in quality-driven policy is mainly due to a welter of reports on severe malpractice being exposed within health and social care. Examples of such reports include those by the Department of Health (DH 2002a, DH 2002b), the Francis Report (2013) and the Department of Health's response to Winterbourne View Hospital (DH 2012). Recent uncovering of malpractice has facilitated changes, based on the implementation of new policy. The evolution of adult safeguarding mirrors what has happened in child protection, in which reactive government policy changes have been made in the light of often heinous abuse and subsequent pressure to reform (Baeza 2011).

In the early 2000s, the notion of 'protecting vulnerable adults' entered the popular lexicon. However, this term has now, almost universally, been replaced by 'safeguarding adults', which will also be used in the rest of this chapter. In Scotland, however, the term 'protecting vulnerable adults' remains topical (Mandelstam 2009). In 2014, a welcome consultation document set out proposals for the development of a new, clear and specific criminal offence of ill treatment or wilful neglect of patients and service users (DH 2014).

Reflective questions

- Reflect on the thoughts you have had, and the judgements you have made, while reading this chapter so far. How have you felt about what you have read?
- What moral and ethical issues has the text raised for you, personally and professionally?
- Consider the social (macro), organisational (meso) and individual (micro) factors that contextualised *why* these abusive acts occurred. What measures have been put in place to address these?
- Reflect on your own personal experience – have you observed or been subject to abusive acts, either in your workplace or in your personal experience of health and social care? If so, how did you respond? How did you feel about the abuse? What, if anything, could you do differently in the future?

Who are vulnerable adults?

The terms used in the process of protection have evolved and this has impacted on who needs protection. 'Safeguarding adults' suggests that those who are deemed to be vulnerable to ill treatment need to be protected from significant others. Perhaps you have a notion of who can be termed a 'vulnerable adult'? It is important to establish how to define a vulnerable individual. Children are perhaps more easily defined by means of their age. The *United Nations Convention on the Rights of a Child* is chronologically specific, defining a child as someone who is under 18 years (Unicef 1989). However, a vulnerable adult is defined as an adult who needs to access health or social care services because of perceived condition-based vulnerability. A vulnerable adult can therefore be seen as 'A person who is or may be in need of community care services by reason of mental or other disability, age or illness; and who is or may be unable to take care of him or herself' (Adult Social Care Statistics Team, Health and Social Care Information Centre 2014).

This definition has been broadened as a result of statutory guidance designed to support local authorities, and the definition of a vulnerable adult has been refined through the description of the safeguarding duties expected of local authority workers. In chapter 14.2 of the Care Act (2014), these safeguarding duties apply in the case of an adult who:

- has needs for care and support
- is experiencing, or is at risk of, abuse or neglect
- as a result of those care and support needs, is unable to protect themselves from either the risk of, or the experience of, abuse or neglect.

This definition describes a service user who is vulnerable in terms of a perceived need to use health or social care services, and whose vulnerability, and incapacity to protect themselves, places them at risk of abuse.

What does adult vulnerability mean in practice?
The legacy of the Francis Report

The conclusion to the report emphasised that at Mid Staffordshire NHS Foundation Trust individual stories of neglect and harm resonated with people's experiences elsewhere in the NHS (DH 2015). This meant that vulnerable adults were abused and at risk across the caring sector.

Consequently, re-establishing the credibility of regulators like the Care Quality Commission (CQC) (England's regulator), and other regulators across the UK, was a critical component of the government response to the inquiry, which sought to establish regulators as trusted and independent agencies that can quickly identify poor care so that effective action is taken. In terms of the CQC, three powerful and independent chief inspectors have been appointed, covering hospitals, general practice and adult social care and thus encompassing a broad spectrum of care. In addition, the CQC's independence has been strengthened via legislation, giving regulators more power to act and drive change. In line with this, the model of inspection used by regulators has been overhauled, moving from a generalist tick-box model to an approach that is informed by experts, patients and staff. This system provides assurance that care is safe, effective, well led, caring and responsive. The critical point here is the notion of a truly *independent regulator* and this is the main issue that readers need to absorb.

Reflective questions

- Who is the regulator in your area of the UK?
- What is their model of inspection?

Furthermore, there has been a drive to ensure that the NHS is open and transparent on key measures of patient safety. The government has placed a new legal duty on all organisations to ensure that when something goes wrong, patients are told about it promptly. Known as the 'duty of candour', this is intended to counteract the legalistic and defensive culture that existed at Mid Staffordshire. In contrast, the 'duty of candour' fosters a culture in which mistakes are acknowledged and learned from (see Chapter 1 for more on this).

Professional regulators, such as the Nursing and Midwifery Council (NMC), are placing consistent responsibilities on health professionals so that action can be taken when they are not candid about errors with their patients (NMC 2015). This professional accountability is being reinforced through the introduction of the role of the 'responsible clinician'. As a result, many hospitals and care providers are now participating in the 'Name above the Bed' initiative, so that patients know who is in charge of their case, and who is accountable for their care and responsible for ensuring continuity of care (Guardian 2014). These changes have been made in the context of a far-reaching programme to open up the NHS.

Reflective questions

- Who is a 'vulnerable adult' and how can you be assured that you would recognise someone who was vulnerable in your everyday practice?
- Who are the regulators in your area of practice? What do they expect of you and the organisation you work in? How do they regulate your practice?
- What is the 'duty of candour' and how does it impact on your practice?

Recent statutory guidance

As a result of recent policy developments, albeit as a reaction to disturbing disclosures, new practitioners (and indeed all health and social care workers irrespective of experience) can access clear guidance to support their practice from a range of sources designed to deliver safe care to vulnerable adults. In 2000 the Department of Health published *No Secrets: Guidance on developing and implementing multi-agency policies and procedures to protect vulnerable adults from abuse*, targeted primarily at local social services concerned with protecting vulnerable adults from abuse. This was superseded by the Care Act (2014) and the Social Services and Well Being (Wales) Act (2014). The aim now is to prevent abuse before it occurs. However, if the preventative strategy fails, agencies should ensure that robust procedures are in place for dealing with abuse. The circumstances in which harm and exploitation occur are known to be extremely diverse, as is membership of the at-risk group; action to respond to this in local situations therefore needs to be clear (meaning that it can be easily understood and put into place).

Prevention takes place through a scheme designed to protect the vulnerable under a rigorous vetting and barring system. The Safeguarding Vulnerable Groups Act (2006) proactively safeguards vulnerable adults. The current legislation was enacted as a result of the supposed systemic shortcomings of previous schemes, such as those identified in the *Bichard Inquiry Report* (2004), which exposed failures in the prevailing system.

The Safeguarding Vulnerable Groups Act (2006) aims to minimise the risk to these groups posed by people who, through working or volunteering in the sector, wish to harm them. It does so by vetting and barring unsuitable individuals from such work. If a person satisfies criteria relating to barred activity, they are included on the Police National Computer barred list.

Regarding those who *are* allowed to work with vulnerable adults, the Care Act (2014) section 14.7 provides unequivocal statutory guidance:

> Safeguarding means protecting an adult's right to live in safety, free from abuse and neglect. It is about people and organisations working together to prevent and stop both the risks and experience of abuse or neglect, while at the same time making sure that the adult's well-being is promoted including, where appropriate, having regard to their views, wishes, feelings and beliefs in deciding on any action.

This guidance sets out these duties as an aspirational philosophy, reflecting the personal wishes of the individual who is in need of safeguarding. Essentially, it places a duty upon the practitioner to work in harmony with significant others involved in the care of the adult – both to prevent exposure to risk of abuse and, if abuse is uncovered, to terminate it.

This has clear links to the Mental Capacity Act (2005), which guides health and social care professionals to ensure that adults' views are expressed within their care plans whilst safeguarding them. The Mental Capacity Act's key tenets emphasise individuals' presumed capacity to make decisions unless proven otherwise, at which point the support needed is given. Anything done for someone without capacity must be done in their best interest and should restrict their freedoms as little as possible. When safeguarding, you should therefore be aware of the urgent need to support adults with capacity to make decisions about their care, as noted in section 14 of the Care Act (2014): 'safeguard adults in a way that supports them in making choices and having control about how they want to live'. Safeguarding must be ethically informed by the Mental Capacity Act (2005), which is based on the precept that people have the right to make choices and decisions about their care. This is a central tenet of everyday health and social care practice.

The aims of adult safeguarding, as encapsulated by the Care Act (2014), may therefore be summarised as, where possible, stopping risk, preventing harm and reducing risk. To achieve these aims, it is important to ensure that everyone (both individuals and organisations) is clear about their roles and responsibilities and creates strong multi-agency partnerships to provide effective prevention/responses to abuse. The Care Act (2014) stresses that one should enable access to mainstream community resources that can reduce the social and physical isolation which, in itself, may increase the risk of abuse. It is also stressed that responses to safeguarding concerns should be clear and timely.

A set of key principles underpin all adult safeguarding work (DH 2011) as follows:

- Empowerment is important so that individuals are supported to make decisions and are aware of the likely outcomes of those decisions.
- Prevention requires action to be taken to prevent something occurring; it also requires the provision of easily understood information about what abuse is, how to recognise signs of abuse, and what to do to seek help.
- Proportionality means responding in the least intrusive manner to the risk presented.
- Protection is emphasised for those in greatest need.
- Partnerships should be sought by services working with their communities to provide local solutions. Communities have a part to play in preventing, detecting and reporting neglect and abuse.
- Accountability and transparency are vital in delivering safeguarding.

The CQC (2016) imposes an organisational duty to safeguard vulnerable adults. They emphasise the importance of outcomes through safeguarding. For the CQC, outcomes are seen as promoting well-being and preventing abuse from happening in the first place, ensuring the safety and well-being of those who have been the subject of abuse, taking action against those who are deemed responsible for abuse or neglect, and finally learning lessons and making changes that could prevent similar abuses happening in the future. Regulators in other parts of the UK share similar principles. The *NHS 'Speaking up' Charter* (DH & Poulter 2012), for example, is supported by many professional bodies; this encourages staff to raise concerns about patient care and be fully supported in so doing (Chartered Society of Physiotherapy 2012).

Reflective questions

- What are the aims and key principles of safeguarding vulnerable adults and how do these affect your practice?
- In your area of practice, what principles does the regulator impose in terms of safeguarding vulnerable adults and how do these impact on what you do on a daily basis?
- How does the *'Speaking up' Charter* impact on your workplace and your responsibilities in caring for vulnerable adults?
- Consider how you would 'speak up' or raise concerns, if you had to, in your workplace. What are the barriers, issues or concerns that worry you about this?

The Health and Care Professions Council (HCPC) and the duty to care

If you are a student or registered allied health professional, you should be familiar with the HCPC codes regarding conduct and ethics (HCPC 2016a & 2016b) and should abide by them. Other professional groups will be subject to similar codes – for example, that of the NMC (2015). There is advice in the HCPC's *Guidance on conduct and ethics for students* (HCPC 2016a) that practitioners access a structure to support their safeguarding work. Its main precepts, which enhance your safeguarding duties, are listed below. These principles apply generally to all health and social care practitioners but you are also urged to reflect on the specifics of your own professional and/or organisational guidance:

- Service users' privacy/dignity must be respected by working in partnership with them, and encouraging them to make informed decisions about their care.
- You must not discriminate against service users, by allowing your personal views to affect the care you provide.
- Polite and considerate communication is encouraged and you should ensure that arrangements are made to meet service users' communication needs.
- It is important to work within your skills base by only practising in the areas for which you have appropriate knowledge, skills and experience; refer a service user to another practitioner if the care, treatment or other services they need are beyond your scope of practice. You are encouraged to delegate appropriately and monitor that work once delegated.
- You are also encouraged to respect confidentiality and disclose confidential information only if you have permission, the law allows it and it is in the service user's best interests.

- Equally, you must take all reasonable steps to reduce the risk of harm to service users, carers and colleagues, ensuring that the safety of a service user is not at risk. Safety concerns linked to the well-being of service users should be reported. You must make sure that you always place the safety and well-being of service users before any professional or other (e.g. organisational or team) loyalties (see also Chapter 13).
- When something has gone wrong with the care, treatment or other services that you provide, openness with service users and other carers is required. You have a duty to inform service users that something has gone wrong and to instigate action to put matters right, ensuring that service users receive a full and prompt explanation of what happened.
- You must support service users and carers who want to raise concerns about the care or treatment they have received or witnessed, and give a helpful and honest response to anyone who complains about the care, treatment or other services they have received.
- Your conduct should justify the public's trust and confidence in you and your profession, and you must always be honest about your experience, qualifications and skills.
- You must inform your professional organisation and employer if you are cautioned by the police or charged with/found guilty of a criminal offence; or another organisation responsible for regulating a health or social care profession has taken action against you; or you have had any restriction placed on your practice; or you have been suspended or dismissed by an employer, because of concerns about your conduct or competence. Finally, you should cooperate with any investigation into your competence.

Profession-specific ethical codes of practice

Your profession's ethical code of practice will always state that it is incumbent upon you to behave in an ethical manner to uphold the value base of the profession. Additionally, it is important to recognise that, as a health and social care professional, you have a responsibility to pass on any concerns about abuse of vulnerable adults as a corollary of your safeguarding duties (Chartered Society of Physiotherapy 2012). Indeed, failure to pass on such concerns may breach the ethical code of conduct associated with your particular health and social care profession (see, for example, College of Occupational Therapists 2015 and Society of Radiographers 2016). Likewise, the professional Code for nurses and midwives (NMC 2015, 16.5/6) tells you not to:

> obstruct, intimidate, victimise or in any way hinder a colleague, member of staff, person you care for or member of the public who wants to raise a concern, and

protect anyone you have management responsibility for from any harm, detriment, victimisation or unwarranted treatment after a concern is raised.

This is a clear endorsement of your duty to raise concerns (previously known as 'whistleblowing') from within the profession, when you have concerns about a colleague's professionalism.

Conclusion

Perhaps the history of safeguarding adults is one that is about to be written. Its emergence is contemporary and, as has been intimated, multifaceted. However, its evolution and success will be influenced hereafter by the activities of new practitioners who have an emerging structure to scaffold their caring duties and an enduring duty to uphold the varied ethical and moral precepts of their professional codes. Fundamentally, this means you must ensure that people are protected from harm, abuse and neglect at all times and that their health, well-being and human rights are paramount in your practice and, indeed, in your everyday life.

Reflective questions

- What is your duty of care and how does it match your own ethical and moral principles?
- How does your professional code of ethics guide you in terms of your responsibilities in safeguarding vulnerable adults?
- If different, how does your registering body guide you in terms of safeguarding vulnerable adults?
- Consider the challenges (if any) presented by your implementation of these codes in your practice?
- Consider the ethical dilemmas you might experience in terms of raising concerns about colleagues, and identify the process in your own organisation that would assist you in raising these concerns. Remember that we all have a legal and moral obligation to protect vulnerable people and the public at large. This must be your priority.

References

Adult Social Care Statistics Team, Health and Social Care Information Centre. (2014). *Abuse of Vulnerable Adults in England 2012–13, Final Report, Experimental Statistics.* Health and Social Information Centre. http://www.hscic.gov.uk/catalogue/PUB13499/abus-vuln-adul-eng-12-13-fin-rep.pdf (last accessed 17.12.2016).

Baker, A.A. (1975). Granny battering. *Modern Geriatrics.* **5**, 20–24.

BBC News (2014). *Hillcroft nursing home staff sentenced for resident abuse.* 24.01.2014. http://www.bbc.co.uk/news/uk-england-lancashire-25676842 (last accessed on 8.4.2016).

Baeza, S. (2011). 'Learning from safeguarding children' in A. Mantell & T. Scragg (eds). *Safeguarding Adults in Social Work.* 2nd edn. Exeter: Learning Matters Ltd.

Bichard, M. (2004). *Bichard Inquiry Report.* http://dera.ioe.ac.uk/6394/1/report.pdf (last accessed 15.6.2016).

Bloch, S. & Singh, B.S. (1999). *Understanding Troubled Minds: A Guide to Mental Illness and Its Treatment.* New York: New York University Press.

Care Act (2014). http://www.legislation.gov.uk/ukpga/2014/23/contents/enacted (last accessed 17.12.2016).

Care Quality Commission (CQC) (2015) *Using Surveillance. Information for providers of health and social care on using surveillance to monitor services.* London: CQC.

Care Quality Commission (CQC) (2016). *Safeguarding Adults,* available at: http://www.cqc.org.uk/ (last accessed 16.06.2016).,

Chartered Society of Physiotherapy (2012). *CSP backs new whistle-blowing charter.* http://www.csp.org.uk/news/2012/10/17/csp-backs-new-whistle-blowing-charter (last accessed 17.12.2016).

College of Occupational Therapists (2015). *Code of Ethics and Professional Conduct.* London: College of Occupational Therapists.

Community Care (2007). *Learning difficulties residential home scandals: the inside story and lessons from Longcare and Cornwall. Community Care.* http://www.communitycare.co.uk/2007/01/10/learning-difficulties-residential-home-scandals-the-inside-story-and-lessons-from-longcare-and-cornwall/#.UoPuhPIT6UM (last accessed 17.12.2016).

Department of Health (DH) (1971). *Better Services for the Mentally Handicapped.* White Paper. London: DH.

Department of Health (DH) (2000). *No secrets: Guidance on Developing and Implementing Multi-Agency Policies and Procedures to Protect Vulnerable Adults from Abuse.* London: DH.

Department of Health (DH) (2002a). *The Shipman Inquiry Safeguarding Patients: Lessons from the Past – Proposals for the Future.* London: The Stationery Office.

Department of Health (DH) (2002b). *Learning from Bristol: the Department of Health Response to the Report of the Public Inquiry into Children's Heart Surgery at the Bristol Royal Infirmary 1984–1995.* London: The Stationery Office.

Department of Health (DH) (2011). *Statement of Government Policy on Adult Safeguarding.* https://www.gov.uk/government/uploads/system/uploads/attachment_data/file/215591/dh_126770.pdf (last accessed on 17.12.2016).

Department of Health (DH) (2012). *Transforming Care: A National Response to Winterbourne View Hospital. Department of Health Review Final Report.* London: DH.

Department of Health (DH) (2014). *New Offence of Wilful Treatment or Neglect Consultation Document.* https://www.gov.uk/government/consultations/ill-treatment-or-wilful-neglect-in-health-and-social-care (last accessed 9.9.2017).

Department of Health (DH) (2015). *Culture change in the NHS: Applying the lessons of the Francis Inquiries.* London: DH.

Department of Health & Poulter, D. (2012). *'Speaking up' Charter encourages staff to raise concerns.* https://www.gov.uk/government/news/speaking-up-charter-encourages-staff-to-raise-concerns. (last accessed 17.12.2016).

Department of Health and Social Security (DHSS) (1969). *Report on Ely Hospital.* London: HMSO.

Department of Health & Tomlinson, D. (1993). *SSI Practice Guidelines. No longer afraid: the safeguard of older people in domestic settings.* London: The Stationery Office.

Donna Ockenden Ltd. (2014). *External Investigation into Care and Treatment of Patients at Tawel Fan Ward, Ablett Acute Mental Health Unit Glan Clwyd Hospital.* http://www.wales.nhs.uk/sitesplus/documents/861/tawel_fan_ward_ockenden_internet.pdf (last accessed 18.12.2016).

Francis, R. (2013). *Report of the Mid Staffordshire NHS Foundation Trust Public Inquiry.* http://www.midstaffspublicinquiry.com/sites/default/files/report/Volume%201.pdf (last accessed 8.4.15).

Griffith, R. (2015). Safeguarding vulnerable adults. *British Journal of Nursing.* **24** (13), 708–709.

Guardian (2014). *Hospital patients 'should have a doctor's name above the bed'.* https://www.theguardian.com/society/2014/jun/13/hospital-patients-named-doctor-medics (last accessed 18.12.2016).

Health and Care Professions Council (HCPC) (2016a). *Guidance on conduct and ethics for students.* London: HCPC.

Health and Care Professions Council (HCPC) (2016b). *Standards on conduct, performance and ethics.* London: HCPC.

Mandelstam, M. (2009). *Safeguarding Vulnerable Adults and the Law.* London: Jessica Kingsley.

McCreadie, C. (2008) From granny battering to elder abuse: a critique of U.K. writing, 1975–1992. *Journal of Elder Abuse and Neglect.* **5** (2), 7–25.

Mental Capacity Act (2005). http://www.legislation.gov.uk/ukpga/2005/9/contents (last accessed 17.12.2016).

Miller, J. (2008). 'Clinical effectiveness skills in practice' in E. Duncan (ed.) *Skills for Practice in Occupational Therapy.* Edinburgh: Churchill Livingstone, Elsevier.

Nursing and Midwifery Council (NMC) (2015). *The Code: Professional standards of practice and behaviour for nurses and midwives.* London: NMC.

Richardson, V. (2014). Safeguarding adults. *Journal of Perioperative Practice.* **24** (5), 118–20.

Safeguarding Vulnerable Groups Act (2006). http://www.legislation.gov.uk/ukpga/2006/47/notes/division/2 (last accessed 15.6.2106).

Social Services and Well Being (Wales) Act (2014). http://www.legislation.gov.uk/anaw/2014/4/pdfs/anaw_20140004_en.pdf (last accessed 17.12.2016).

Society of Radiographers (2016). *Code of Professional Conduct.* http://www.sor.org/learning/document-library/code-professional-conduct/statements-professional-conduct (last accessed 15.06.2016).

Sutton, C. (1992). *Confronting Elder Abuse: An SSI London Region Survey.* Great Britain: Social Services Inspectorate, Great Britain: Department of Health, London: The Stationery Office.

Unicef (1989). *The United Nations Convention on the Rights of a Child.* London: Unicef UK. https://downloads.unicef.org.uk/wp-content/uploads/2010/05/UNCRC_united_nations_convention_on_the_rights_of_the_child.pdf (last accessed 9.9.2017).

Chapter 12
Safeguarding children

Ian Smith

Learning outcomes
By the end of this chapter you will be able to:
- Reflect on the evolution and background of child protection and understand why it developed in the UK
- Explain what is meant by 'safeguarding' children and understand various types of abuse, including female genital mutilation (FGM)
- Show an understanding of the guidance and legislation relevant to safeguarding children and consider its influence on your ethical and moral principles, both as a practitioner and an individual
- Consider how, as a future and/or developing practitioner, this guidance and legislation impacts on your individual practice, your profession and your organisation and understand what actions you need to take when a concern has been identified.

Introduction
Protecting children and young people from harm needs to be high on the agenda for all health and social care professionals and is often considered to be one of the most challenging areas of practice. All staff have a responsibility to handle the safeguarding of children effectively, to minimise the risk of harm to children. They must also know what to do when they have a concern.

This chapter will explore the various pieces of legislation and guidance that concern the elements of safeguarding children. It will identify how this legislation and guidance impacts on individual practitioners and health and social care organisational responsibilities. The historical background will also be explored, highlighting high-profile child safeguarding incidents that influenced change. In order to contextualise discussions, the following issues will be covered:

- The terms 'child protection' and 'child in need' will be defined, and the specific differences and actions required will be described.
- The different categories of abuse will be explained, highlighting indicators of the various types. Specific information on FGM will be given and the categories explained, together with background information on FGM. Further expansion of registered practitioners' responsibilities for FGM will be highlighted and the potential impact on registration clarified.
- Children's rights will be explored specifically around the United Nations Convention on the Rights of the Child (United Nations 1989) and what this actually means in practice.
- The levels of training required by various grades of staff will be discussed and the required level of training highlighted.
- Professional optimism and professional curiosity will be explained, whilst differentiating between the two, and identifying best practice in order to safeguard children and young people.
- Finally, the actions that need to be taken by individual practitioners and organisations will be discussed.

Evolution and history of child protection

Child protection can be dated back to the eighteenth-century industrial revolution, which was an age of steam, coal, canals and factories. The invention of new machinery and technology replaced water and animal power with steam power, and made mass production possible. The coal, steam and iron era allowed larger-scale manufacturing of many products (Manolopoulou 2009). These advances would change the nature of Britain's economy, and the way children were perceived and treated, for ever.

Greater production created a need for more workers, and many textile factories turned to child labour to plug this gap (Levene 2010). Orphans, known as 'pauper apprentices', were utilised but not paid for their services, receiving only food and basic shelter in return for their labour (Levene 2010). These factories were dangerous, with many injuries and deaths occurring (National Archives 2016). Using children in this way can be seen as the first known account of child exploitation.

Arguably the first law that considered child protection was the Health and Morals of Apprentices Act (1802). This aimed to reduce the exploitation of children in factories (Levene 2010). This was followed by many other laws that protected children from dangerous and exploitative activities in mines and factories (Nardinelli 1980). Thus the eighteenth and nineteenth centuries not only saw the evolution of the industrial revolution but also the beginning of child protection, leading to improvements in children's education, health and welfare.

After years of lobbying by the founders of the National Society for the Prevention of Cruelty to Children (NSPCC), the first Act of Parliament for the prevention of cruelty to children was passed – the Prevention of Cruelty to, and Protection of, Children Act (1889), also known as the Children's Charter (NSPCC 2011). Various other laws were developed to help protect children over the following years. In 1933, the Children and Young Persons Act (1933) brought together all existing child protection law into a single piece of legislation.

However, on 9 January 1945 a child called Dennis O'Neill died, aged 13. He was undernourished, thin and wasted, with septic ulcers on his feet, and his legs were severely chapped. Dennis and his brother Terence, who survived, were fed bread and butter and tea by their foster carers. They were also regularly beaten (O'Neill 2010). Following Dennis O'Neill's death, the Children Act (1948) was passed.

Despite this legislation, children continued to die at the hands of their carers, and the deaths of four-year-old Jasmine Beckford, Kimberley Carlisle (also aged four) and 16-month-old Doreen Mason (amongst many others) prompted a review of child protection law. As a result of these ongoing deaths, the Children Act (1989) was developed. This is a significant piece of child protection legislation, giving every child the right to protection from abuse and exploitation. The Act placed a duty on every local authority to provide appropriate services for children in need and to ensure that child protection measures are in place (Welsh Assembly Government 2006). It also placed a duty on all regulated authorities to co-operate in safeguarding and promote the welfare of children. This regulation places a responsibility on health care workers, as health care is a regulated authority.

In the same year as the Children Act (1989), the United Nations Convention on the Rights of the Child (UNCRC) (United Nations 1989) was established. This international agreement protects the rights of children, providing a child-centred framework for the development of children's services. It places a responsibility on governments to embrace the UNCRC and ensures that children's voices are heard, they are protected from harmful situations and suitable provision is made to meet their needs. The UNCRC took 30 years to develop, was completed in 1989 and was accepted by all the United Nation states – except Somalia and the USA. Somalia did not have a stable government that could ratify the treaty and, although the USA *did* endorse the principles, it believed that the Convention would hinder its constitutional rights (Blanchfield 2013). Even though the UK ratified the UNCRC in 1991, this did not prevent further child deaths through abuse, which led to further legislation being developed.

This brings us into the twenty-first century, at which point another significant child death took place. Victoria Climbié was an eight-year-old child brought to this country from the Ivory Coast via France by her great-aunt. On 25 February 2000, Victoria died of hypothermia and multiple organ failure. She had sustained 128 horrific injuries to her body, after suffering months of abuse and neglect at the hands of her great-aunt and her aunt's boyfriend. Following her death, a public inquiry was set up, chaired by Lord Laming. This inquiry found that there had been 12 key opportunities for professionals to intervene to safeguard Victoria, none of which were considered to require any great skill (Laming 2003). Subsequently, the inquiry presented no fewer than 108 recommendations to improve practice across many different professional disciplines (Laming 2003).

The untimely and brutal death of Victoria Climbié and the ensuing inquiry were instrumental in the development of the Children Act (2004). Therefore, in some ways, it could be said that Victoria's short life and tragic death helped save many other children. The Children Act (2004) made amendments to the Children Act (1989). It sought to emphasise the importance of interagency work and co-operation in meeting the needs of children, to ensure that children's views were taken into account and represented and to improve outcomes for all children, including those categorised as 'in need' under the Children Act (1989). It was aimed at focusing services more effectively around the needs of children, young people and families. The Children Act (2004) can be considered a turning point in child protection as it signalled a demonstrable shift in approach, from purely child protection to one of prevention. It formed Statutory Local Safeguarding Children Boards (LSCBs) in England and Wales, providing support for health and social care professionals in working together and sharing information to identify difficulties and making regulatory authorities accountable for their actions or inactions. This also places a responsibility on individual practitioners to ensure that children are protected from harm.

Reflective questions

- Reflecting on what you have read so far, what do you think about the social and cultural factors shaping the development of safeguarding children both in the UK and globally?
- How do you feel, ethically and morally, about these factors?

- Are you aware of any other atrocities perpetrated on children since the Climbié case? If so, what are your thoughts on why these terrible events are continuing to occur in contemporary society?
- What do you think society should do to value children differently and both respect them and hear their voices?

Defining key terms

Section 17 of the Children Act (1989) defines a child as being legally 'in need' if:

- they are unlikely to achieve or maintain or have the opportunity to achieve or maintain a reasonable standard of health or development without provision of services from the Local Authority
- their health or development is likely to be significantly impaired, or further impaired, without the provision of services from the Local Authority
- they have a disability.

Moreover, Section 47 of the Children Act (1989) states that 'child protection' is the process of protecting individual children who have been identified as either suffering, or likely to suffer, significant harm as a result of abuse or neglect. It involves measures and structures designed to prevent and respond to abuse and neglect.

The categories of abuse are defined by the NSPCC as 'physical', 'emotional', 'sexual' and 'neglect'. Children can be placed on the child protection register under one or a combination of these types of abuse.

Physical abuse

Physical abuse is defined as deliberately hurting a child, causing injuries such as bruises, fractures, burns or cuts; violence is used, including being hit, kicked, poisoned, burned, slapped or having objects thrown at them; shaking babies can cause non-accidental head injuries. Parents or carers may make up or cause the symptoms of illness to their child, by making the child unwell. This is known as 'fabricated' or 'induced' illness (previously often referred to as 'Munchausen by Proxy syndrome').

Emotional abuse

Emotional abuse is the persistent emotional ill treatment of a child so as to cause severe and persistent adverse effects on the child's emotional development and well-being. Emotional abuse can involve deliberately trying to scare or humiliate a child, isolating or ignoring them or making them feel unloved.

Sexual abuse

Sexual abuse involves forcing or enticing a child or young person to take part in sexual activities, whether or not the child is aware of what is happening. This does not necessarily have to involve physical contact; it can also occur online, through video filming or photography or through voyeurism.

Child sexual exploitation (CSE) is a type of sexual abuse where children or young people are tricked or coerced into sexual relationships for which they receive some form of payment. For instance, they might be invited to parties and given drugs, alcohol, gifts or money (Kirtley 2013).

Neglect

Neglect is the persistent failure to meet basic physical and/or psychological needs, which is likely to result in the serious impairment of the child's health and development. This is the most common form of abuse – there are more children on the child protection register for neglect than for any other form of abuse.

Female genital mutilation

Female genital mutilation (FGM) is a specific type of abuse. Although it is not an official category of abuse according to the child protection register, it is undoubtedly physical and sexual abuse and arguably emotional abuse (UNICEF 2013). The scale of the problem is enormous; somewhere between 100 and 140 million women and girls globally are believed to have undergone FGM (UNICEF 2013). The World Health Organisation (WHO 2010) suggests that FGM is a practice that is prevalent in around 29 different countries in Sub-Saharan Africa, from the Atlantic coast to the Horn of Africa, North-East Africa, Iraq and Yemen. However, girls all over the world are at risk of FGM, many travelling from the country they live in to traditional homelands to undergo FGM (Griffith & Tengnah 2009). The Royal College of Midwives and other key bodies believe that FGM is also practised across Europe (Royal College of Midwives *et al.* 2013).

FGM can be described as the cutting and alteration of the female genitalia for non-clinical reasons. It is practised predominantly on infants, but also on girls, adolescents and sometimes adults (UNICEF 2013). It is often carried out by members of the immediate or extended family. The practice is also known as female circumcision and FGM/C (female genital mutilation/cutting) (WHO 2010). The terms 'cutting' and 'mutilation' emphasise that the practice is an abhorrent violation of the rights of women and girls.

There are four types of FGM. The World Health Organisation (2010), together with many other organisations, describes them as follows:

- The first type is clitorectomy, which is when there is an excision of the skin surrounding the clitoris. It may include the partial or total excision of clitoris, also known as *sunna*.
- The second is the excision of the clitoris with total or partial excision of the labia minora.

- Type three is known as infibulation. This involves excision of the entire clitoris and some or all of the labia minora. Incisions are then made in the outer folds of skin surrounding the vulva, the labia majora. The raw surfaces of the labia are then stitched together in order to cover the opening of the vagina and the urethra, leaving a small posterior opening that is only large enough to accommodate urinary and menstrual blood flow.
- The fourth type involves a variety of procedures that damages the female genitalia. This can include: pricking, piercing, stretching; incisions of the clitoris and/or the labia; cauterisation of the clitoris and/or surrounding tissues by burning; making incisions to the vaginal wall; scraping or cutting of the vagina; or using herbs or other corrosive substances in the vagina in order to scar and/or narrow the vagina (WHO 2010). This is undoubtedly an act of child abuse when performed on a child.

It is important that when abuse or neglect is identified, or even suspected, that people share their concerns. Nearly every review into the death of a child has identified 'missed opportunities' where sharing of information could or should have protected that child. It's therefore vital to know what your responsibilities are, and what should be done (Brandon *et al.* 2008). Although strangers can abuse children, it should be remembered that they are more commonly abused by a family member or someone known to them (NSPCC 2009). This is a critical point for health and social care practitioners to bear in mind, as abuse may be taking place within the family network and/or home of a family with whom you work. To support growing concerns about reporting possible cases of FGM, several guidelines have recently been produced. These include statutory guidance found in the *Multi-agency Statutory Guidance on Female Genital Mutilation* (HM Government 2016) and guidance on practice found in the *FGM Safeguarding and Risk Assessment: A Quick Guide for Health Professionals* (DH 2017a) and the associated FGM Safeguarding Pathway (DH 2017b).

Reflective questions

- What were your thoughts and how did you feel when reading about children needing 'protection', being 'in need', or when you read about the definitions of abuse?
- What kind of signs and symptoms do you think you may notice if a child is being abused?
- How might you recognise some of the more 'hidden' types of abuse (such as emotional, sexual or FGM)?

Responsibilities placed on organisations and practitioners

The Children Act (1989 and 2004) and the Serious Crimes Act (2015) place statutory responsibilities on both organisations and individual health care practitioners. Organisations and individuals also have to embrace the fundamental principles of the UNCRC (1989). In practice, this means that health care organisations have to ensure that they discharge their functions (including any services they contract out to others) while having due regard to the need to safeguard and promote the welfare of children. They have to ensure that the appropriate resources are in place to meet their obligations under the Children Act (2004) (Welsh Assembly Government 2006). This includes safe recruitment and retention of staff, providing appropriate training for staff, having clear lines of accountability within the organisation, having an appropriate strategic structure and appropriate policies in place to ensure effective and appropriate information sharing. The UNCRC gives organisations responsibility for ensuring that their practices promote participation, provision and protection for children and young people when developing policies and practices that impact upon a child.

The legislation also imposes responsibilities on individual health care practitioners to ensure that they also promote the safety and well-being of children in their day-to-day practice, protecting children from abuse, neglect and harm. As a health care practitioner, you will have to ensure that you do not do anything that will bring harm to children (or fail to do something that will protect them). The principles ensuring the safety of children extend outside the working environment and into everyday life. This, together with safe and effective working practices, means that practitioners are duty-bound to ensure that they share any suspected or identified concerns with appropriate line managers and local authorities, who have a legislative duty to protect children. There are some circumstances that will require you to share information directly with the police (Brandon *et al.* 2008).

Training

All staff who work with or alongside children have to have safeguarding training commensurate with their roles and responsibilities. *Safeguarding Children and Young people: Roles and Competences for Health Care Staff: The Intercollegiate Document* sets out a specific training framework for health care staff, depending on their particular roles and responsibilities, establishing a set of knowledge, skills, attitudes and values required to ensure safe and effective practice (Royal College of Paediatrics and Child Health 2014). The framework consists of five levels, each increasing in content and core competencies:

- Level 1 is aimed at all staff working in health care settings.
- Level 2 is for all clinical and non-clinical staff who have contact with children, young people and/or their parents/carers.
- Level 3 is for clinical staff working with children, young people and/or their parents/carers and may contribute to assessing, planning, intervening and evaluating the needs of a child or young person and parenting capacity where there are safeguarding/child protection concerns.
- Level 4 is aimed at specialist roles, e.g. named professionals.
- Level 5 is for specialist roles such as designated professionals.

The health care organisation is responsible for ensuring that their staff have the appropriate training for their role, based on the above information.

What to do in practice

Each organisation should have a safeguarding children policy and procedure. It is important that these procedures are followed appropriately. They will give you guidance on what to do if you identify a concern. Over the years, several serious case reviews have identified poor practices, with missed opportunities to share information that could have helped protect children (Brandon *et al.* 2008).

If you have identified an actual or potential concern, no matter how small it appears, it is vital that you share that concern appropriately. If the child is in immediate danger, the police should be informed so that they can take appropriate action. If there is no immediate danger, you should discuss your concerns with your supervisor, line manager or directly with the appropriate local authority (Department of Health 2012). In addition to this, the Serious Crimes Act (2015) requires registered health and social care professionals to ensure that they notify the police if they are informed by a girl aged under 18 that an act of FGM has been carried out on her; or if they observe physical signs indicating that FGM has been carried out on a girl under 18 and they do not believe that this was necessary for labour or childbirth, or for the girl's physical or mental health. Failing to comply with this legislation can result in action being taken by governing bodies such as the General Medical Council, Nursing and Midwifery Council and/or the Health and Care Professions Council.

Reflective questions

- What would you do in your practice if you felt a child was in immediate danger?
- How would you share concerns in your organisation?
- How do you feel about sharing such concerns?

- What knowledge, skills, attitudes and values do you possess, in relation to safeguarding? And how do your knowledge, skills, attitudes and values align with those required to ensure safe and effective practice?

The rule of optimism and professional curiosity

There is a tendency for health and social care workers to attempt to rationalise the information put before them in certain situations, with workers focusing on adults' strengths and believing that the adult has the best interests of the child at heart. This phenomenon is frequently known as 'the rule of optimism' (Dingwell, Eekelaar & Murray 2014) and it can result in parents not being challenged sufficiently. An example of this is a baby presenting with injuries at an Emergency Department whose family is part of a culture of drug misuse. The mother is well presented, articulate and described by some staff as 'a lovely girl'. This leads them to accept the information provided by the mother about her level of drug misuse and her ability to care for and protect her children. The causes of the injuries therefore go unchallenged, and the opportunity to share information is missed (Kirtley 2013).

Serious case reviews have concluded that professionals should be prepared to challenge information from parents, carers or other professionals in order to establish the difference between facts, hearsay and opinion. This was certainly the case with Victoria Climbié, when health and social care professionals believed Victoria's aunt's version of events. However, it is not for practitioners to play detective, but to uphold an ethos of 'professional curiosity' (Dingwell, Eekelaar & Murray 2014). Professional curiosity, also known as 'respectful uncertainty', requires health and social care practitioners not just to observe what is being said, but also to be aware of non-verbal clues (such as body language) to ensure that the information being given is actually consistent with the injuries or illness being presented. It is vital to notice small details in presentation, and the way children behave and react, to avoid falling into the trap of professional optimism (Brandon, Bailey & Belderson 2010).

Reflective questions

- Considering your practice and personal experience to date, do you think you may have missed an opportunity to protect a child?
- Can you identify an occasion (at work or in your personal life) when you may have employed the 'rule of optimism', instead of 'professional curiosity' or 'respectful uncertainty'?
- If so, what would you do differently in the future and how can you be sure that you will adopt the correct mindset henceforth in both your practice and personal life?

Conclusion

It is *everybody's* responsibility to safeguard children's welfare – not just managers, supervisors and those specialist people working directly with children. These responsibilities are underpinned by legislation that has been developed over many years. Abuse and neglect comes in many forms and adversely affects the health, development and well-being of children. It is important that health care workers not only exercise their statutory duties but also their moral and ethical duties. We need to adopt professional curiosity, as opposed to professional optimism, and act appropriately by following organisational guidance and sharing information. These actions will help reduce missed opportunities and help protect children.

References

To assist with chronology, the names of relevant monarchs have been noted against Acts of Parliament.

Blanchfield, L. (2013). *The United Nations Convention on the Rights of the Child Congressional Research Service.* https://www.fas.org/sgp/crs/misc/R40484.pdf (last accessed 08.09.2016).

Brandon, M., Bailey, S. & Belderson, P. (2010). *Building on the Learning from Serious Case Reviews: A Two Year Analysis of Child Protection Database Notifications 2007–2009.* Norwich: University of East Anglia.

Brandon, M., Belderson, P., Warren, C., Howe, D., Gardner, R., Dodsworth, J. & Black, J. (2008). *Analysing Child Deaths and Serious Injury Through Abuse and Neglect: What Can We Learn? A Biennial Analysis of Serious Case Reviews 2003–2005.* Nottingham: Department for Children, Schools and Families.

Children Act 1948 (George VI). http://nationalarchives.gov.uk/cabinetpapers/themes/protection-children.htm (last accessed 18.12.2016).

Children Act 1989 (Elizabeth II). London: The Stationery Office.

Children Act 2004 (Elizabeth II). London: The Stationery Office.

Children and Young Persons Act 1933 (George V). http://www.legislation.gov.uk/ukpga/Geo5/23-24/12 (last accessed 18.12.2016).

Department of Health (DH) (2012). *Health Visiting and School Nurse Programme: Supporting Implementation of the New Service Offer No. 5: Safeguarding Children and Young People: Enhancing Professional Practice – Working with Children and Families.* London: DH.

Department of Health (DH) (2017a) *FGM Safeguarding and Risk Assessment: A Quick Guide for Health Professionals.* London: DH.

Department of Health (DH) (2017b) *FGM Safeguarding Pathway.* London: DH.

Dingwell, R., Eekelaar, J. & Murray, T. (2014) *The Protection of Children.* New Orleans: Quid Pro Books.

Griffith, R. & Tengnah, C. (2009). The Female Genital Mutilation Act 2003: an overview for district nurses. *British Journal of Community Nursing.* **14** (2), 86–89.

Health and Morals of Apprentices Act 1802 (George III). London: The Stationery Office.

Kirtley, P. (2013). *'If you Shine a Light You Will Probably Find it' Report of a Grass Roots Survey of Health Professionals with Regard to their Experiences in Dealing with Child Sexual Exploitation.* NWG Network tackling Child Sexual Exploitation. http://www.nhs.uk/aboutNHSChoices/professionals/healthandcareprofessionals/child-sexual-exploitation/Documents/Shine%20a%20Light.pdf (last accessed 18.12.2016).

HM Government (2016). *Multi-agency Statutory Guidance on Female Genital Mutilation.* London: HM Government.

Laming, W.H. (2003). *The Victoria Climbié Inquiry.* London: The Stationery Office.

Levene, A. (2010). Parish apprenticeship and the old poor law in London. *Economic History Review.* **63**, (4), 915–41.

Manolopoulou, A. (2009). *The Industrial Revolution and the Changing Face of Britain.* The British Museum. http://www.britishmuseum.org/research/publications/online_research_catalogues/paper_money/paper_money_of_england__wales/the_industrial_revolution.aspx (last accessed 20.1. 2016).

Nardinelli, C. (1980). Child labour and the Factory Act. *Journal of Economic History.* **14** (4), 739–55.

National Archives (2016). *The Struggle for Democracy: Child Labour.* http://www.nationalarchives.gov.uk/pathways/citizenship/struggle_democracy/childlabour.htm (last accessed 7.8.2016).

National Society for the Prevention of Cruelty to Children (NSPCC) (2009). *Child Protection Fact Sheet: The Definitions and Signs of Child Abuse.* London: NSPCC.

National Society for the Prevention of Cruelty to Children (NSPCC) (2011). *A Pocket History of the NSPCC.* London: NSPCC.

O'Neill, T. (2010). *Someone to Love Us.* London: Harper Element.

Prevention of Cruelty to, and Protection of, Children Act 1889 (Victoria).

Royal College of Midwives, Royal College of Nursing, Royal College of Obstetricians and Gynaecologists, Equality Now and UNITE (2013). *Tackling FGM in the UK: Intercollegiate Recommendations for Identifying, Recording, and Reporting.* London: Royal College of Midwives.

Royal College of Paediatrics and Child Health (2014). *Safeguarding Children and Young people: Roles and Competences for Health Care Staff: The Intercollegiate Document.* London: Royal College of Paediatrics and Child Health.

Serious Crimes Act 2015 (Elizabeth II). London: The Stationery Office.

United Nations (1989). *United Nations Convention on the Rights of the Child (UNCRC).* Geneva: United Nations.

UNICEF (2013). *Female Genital Mutilation/Cutting: A Statistical Overview and Exploration of the Dynamics of Change.* New York: UNICEF.

Welsh Assembly Government (2006). *Safeguarding Children: Working Together Under the Children Act 2004.* Cardiff: Welsh Assembly Government.

World Health Organisation (2010). *Global Strategy to Stop Health Care Providers from Performing Female Genital Mutilation.* Geneva: WHO Press.

Chapter 13

Evidencing caring values in everyday practice

Teena J. Clouston

Learning outcomes

By the end of this chapter you will be able to:

- Describe what 'caring' values are and why they are essential to your everyday practice in health and social care settings
- Understand how the values of staff and organisational cultures can influence the practice of care and compassion in health and social care settings
- Consider how, as a future and/or developing practitioner, you can evidence these values in your everyday practice
- Appreciate why awareness of, and the ability to adapt and change your personal values and interpersonal skills, are important to you as a caring practitioner.

Introduction

The crucial role the workforce plays in ensuring the provision of high-quality, safe health and social care for service users (patients or clients), and indeed the well-being of the staff group as a whole, has been clearly identified in recent reports in the United Kingdom (see Francis 2013 and Andrews 2014 for compelling evidence). Unsurprisingly, in a field known as health and social *care*, there is an expectation that people doing the 'caring' for others, in whatever role they hold (whether they are working in hotel services or as health care practitioners and managers), will do this with due consideration.

At the most basic level, this means noting and responding to the needs of those they care for by meeting not only the basic requirements necessary for survival (e.g.

drinking, feeding, toileting), but also other aspects of Maslow's (1948) hierarchy of needs, such as safety and belonging. Providing safety is necessary, in terms of ensuring medical stability and meeting psychosocial requirements like housing and security; while a sense of belonging includes the notion of trust. This quality is imperative for meeting needs at an interpersonal level, but also lays a foundation for the more altruistic, mutually reciprocal interactions that reflect our shared humanity and lead us to form caring and/or supportive relationships and gain the emotional ability to feel empathy and compassion for others.

In line with this relational and interpersonal aspect of human nature, is the basic assumption that the giving of care will be proffered with the dignity and respect that people, as human beings, should receive and freely give to others. Significantly, whilst these values should be extended to everyone, in all walks of life, in the health and social care arenas they are doubly important: those receiving care can feel vulnerable and be in pain, and therefore require 'care' (in every sense of the word). Of course, care, compassion, empathy, dignity and respect are behaviours we should all exhibit every day but, in order to give a shared understanding of what we mean by these and other 'caring' values, some definitions are given in Table 13.1.

Table 13.1 Defining caring values in health and social care

Values	Meaning in health and social care	Embodied behaviour and practice
Advocacy	This means supporting others by speaking up on their behalf and protecting their rights. In terms of health and social care, there is some debate as to whether or not professionals/practitioners can be objective advocates. However, in terms of human rights and caring values, it is essential: in this context advocacy is linked to *courage* and *being caring*.	Speaking out on behalf of others when there is injustice or people are not being heard; promoting the rights of others and protecting the rights of those who are vulnerable.
Care	This includes being caring and applying a duty of care. In the first instance, this is about meeting personal care needs and enacting a caring approach (i.e. providing whatever is necessary for the welfare and protection of the other person). The duty of care is about ensuring that you *do no harm* (non-maleficence) and in fact *do good* (beneficence).	Meeting personal needs with dignity and respect. This includes taking time to listen and understand concerns, appreciating differing viewpoints and cultures respectfully, dealing with personal care considerately, asking and explaining before doing, being person-centred, attentive and responsive to others, e.g. offering water and taking a person to the toilet when required.

Compassion	A deep and meaningful awareness of the suffering of another, coupled with the wish to relieve it. It is strongly associated with an awareness of psychological, emotional and spiritual concerns.	Seven dimensions associated with compassion are: *attentiveness, listening, confronting, involvement, helping, presence and understanding* (Sinclair et al. 2016).
Courage	To do the right thing; to speak out against injustice.	This is about having the strength to take responsibility for your own judgement; to challenge concerns and speak out or report others ('whistleblow') in order to protect and maintain values; also to innovate and develop practice (Watterson 2013).
Dignity	Treating someone as if they are worthy of merit; recognising they are autonomous and feeling human beings who are worthy of respect (Galloway 2013).	Consider individual preferences in the way that care is delivered; respect individual differences; make the person feel valued in your interactions with them; do not ignore basic care needs and small acts of kindness, e.g. brushing hair and taking a moment to listen and respond meaningfully; consider emotions such as embarrassment, fear, loss of control and autonomy when in hospital settings, where independence is compromised and when intimate and personal care or investigations are carried out.
Empathy	Understanding and emotionally attuning yourself to the feelings and experiences of another; it is also about appreciating the personal meaning of patient's words (Halpern 2003).	Recognising and validating the presence of strong feelings in the care setting (e.g. fear, anger, grief, disappointment); pausing to imagine how the patient might be feeling; stating your perception of the patient's feeling (e.g. 'I can imagine that must be …' or 'It sounds as if you're upset about …'); legitimising that feeling; respecting the patient's effort to cope with their predicament; offering support and partnership (e.g. 'I'm committed to working with you to …' or 'Let's see what we can do together to …') (Platt 1992, cited in Hardee 2003 p. 52).
Integrity	Behaving in a way that ensures you do what is right and responsible at all times. In a professional context, this means evidencing that your ethical and professional standards are enacted and your reputation remains intact.	Being professional in your behaviour and approach, e.g. being honest and open when things go wrong, being true to yourself and others, being genuine and reliable at all times (whether or not others are watching).

Being non-judgemental	Not judging or being judgemental of others in practice or in your personal life.	Recognising and appreciating equality and diversity, celebrating difference, and ensuring that any conscious or unconscious bias you may hold is extinguished or explored and adjusted.
Being person-centred	Having a genuine regard for the person and listening to their wishes so they can live the life they want to live.	Using the 'transcendent lens', i.e. thinking about the effects of your decisions on others, listening and responding genuinely, exhibiting genuine positive regard for the other person, valuing their choices and meeting their personal needs (see pp. 177, 178).
Respect	Having due regard for the feelings and wishes of others.	This could include recognising and taking into account the views and values of others, being mindful of and giving attention to others, respecting confidentiality, privacy and vulnerability or concerns. This is also about facilitating shared decision-making (Coulter & Collins 2011).
Trust	Engendering confidence and creating a bond with others.	Maintaining competence in your skills and fitness to practise, working in the best interests of the patient/client at all times (Calnan & Rowe 2004) and following through on promises made.

When looking over Table 13.1, remember that for those who hold a professional qualification, these ethical frameworks and standards underpin practice, making this expectation of care into a *duty* that must be achieved in order to ensure fitness to practise (see Chapters 11 and 12 for more on the duty of care). It is perhaps surprising, then, that there have been so many recent examples of both individual practitioners and the organisations they work for failing to meet even the most basic needs of their patients/service users. A snapshot of some of the most recent and distressing inquiries is given in Table 13.2. The resulting reports propose an unsettling spectrum of causal factors, ranging from poor practice and criminal behaviour perpetrated by one or more individuals (Clothier 1994, Shipman 2005) to wider, collective and broad-spectrum organisational failure (Andrews 2014, Francis 2013, Haringey 2009, Laming 2003, Winterbourne View 2014, DH 2012a).

Table 13.2 Reports on failings in health and social care

Clothier Inquiry (1994)	• Qualified nurse Beverley Allitt killed four children and attacked nine others. She was found to be suffering from Munchausen Syndrome by Proxy but this was not recognised in her training or subsequent work, despite a history of illness and behavioural problems from childhood. Organisational failures were described in the report, including ineffective ward management and a pervasive lack of interest in care by senior management. • Recommendations made included: increasing the safeguarding procedures for children and support staff to report allegations and raise concerns. The resulting Public Interest Disclosure Act (1998) provided legal support and legislated to prevent whistleblowers being victimised or dismissed. This was updated in 2013 following the Francis Report (Francis 2013). Consider: has this worked? If so, how? If not what is needed?
Shipman Inquiry (Six reports 2002–2005)	• GP Harold Shipman was convicted of murdering 15 patients and forging a will. Later investigations uncovered at least 214 murders (all of older people), committed throughout a career spanning 25 years. His motives for killing, when not for personal financial gain, are unknown. To date, he is the most prolific serial killer in recorded history. • Recommendations included: increasing safeguarding procedures for the public by ensuring checks on qualifications, police checks and increased powers of suspension by employing authorities. Consider: has this worked? If so, how? If not, what is needed?
Laming Report (2003)	• Victoria Climbié was an eight-year-old girl who was tortured and murdered by her guardians whilst being involved with several 'care' agencies, including Social Services, the NHS, schools and the NSPCC. The report highlighted a 'gross failure of the system' (Laming 2003, p.3) and 'widespread organisational malaise' (p.4). • Recommendations included: clear lines of accountability, strong management, who take responsibility and don't 'pass the buck' (p.4) and 'a clear set of values about the role of public service' (p.5), including the public good and protection of vulnerable people. Consider: has this worked? If so, how? If not, what is needed?
Haringey Serious Case Review (Baby P) (2009)	• Peter Connolly (Baby P), a 17-month-old child, died after suffering over 50 injuries in an eight-month period. He was known and considered an active case to multiple agencies including health, social care and the police. Poor communication, limited report writing and inconsistent care were all highlighted as causal to his death. • Recommendations included: a multi-agency review of protocols, communication strategies and action procedures to prevent children being lost in the system. The Laming Report (2009) required an investment in staff (especially social workers) to tackle recruitment and retention issues and to provide extra support, specific training in safeguarding children, guaranteed supervision time and guidelines on maximum workloads. Consider: has this worked? If so, how? If not, what is needed?

Francis Report (2013)	• Inquiries into Mid Staffordshire NHS Foundation Trust found pervasive failure on behalf of the Trust board to address 'an insidious negative culture involving a tolerance of poor standards' (p.3) in order to meet the requirements for foundation trust status and national access targets. 'Appalling care' (p.7), specifically marked in the care of older people, was identified. • Recommendations included putting the needs of patients before anything else, emphasis on shared common values by all, individually and organisationally, and the rigorous scrutiny of standards of care. **Consider**: has this worked? If so, how? If not, what is needed?
Winterbourne View – Time for Change (2014)	• Winterbourne View was a private facility run by Castlebeck Care Ltd. The first report Transforming care (DH 2012a) identified serious abuse, a closed and punitive culture and management failure. Whistleblowers, clients and relatives' concerns were all ignored. The Panorama programme 'Uncover care: Abuse exposed' was the catalyst that brought the case to light. The impact on clients and their families has been profound. • As recommendations from the 2012 report have not been met, so the resulting 2014 report recommends: a 'Charter of Rights' (p. 9) for people with learning disabilities and/or autism that should underpin commissioning, closure of inappropriate institutional inpatient facilities, building capacity of community support and policies to hold organisations and their employees to account for care given. Consider: has this worked? If so, how? If not, what is needed?
Trusted to Care (2014) (The Andrews Report)	• Investigation into the care of older people in Princess of Wales and Neath & Port Talbot Hospitals (ABMU Health Board) highlighted poor professional behaviour, care lacking elements of dignity and respect, lack of suitably qualified or motivated staff, aggressive and/or poor responses to complaints, and problems with organisational strategies of quality and patient safety. • Recommendations included creating a culture that supports staff to: practise professionally, collectively and individually, to work in cohesive teams, to ensure the right staff are there at the right time on a 24/7 basis and to develop a 'psychological contact' (p.3) between the organisation and the staff which 'allows them to shape what ABMU does and how it does it'. Consider: has this worked? If so, how? If not, what is needed?

Whilst, on first reading, these incidents can appear as random occurrences, in fact there is a common thread that ties them all together: they collectively share an organisational cultural context that either ignored or condoned these incidents by driving performance outcomes that were the antithesis of caring values, even when this was noted and concerns were raised.

However you look at this, and whatever excuses you make, this lack of intervention and action to prevent failures and, ultimately, people dying, is astounding. Of course, investigations have been carried out and recommendations made following each and every one of these known incidents; some of the outcomes of these investigations are noted against the respective reports in Table 13.2. However, it is clear from the timeline of these reports (1994 to 2013) that, even though recommendations have been made, failings have continued to happen. Research suggests that this is because, although solutions are considered, they are not fully implemented or acculturated into everyday organisational practice (Paton & McCalman 2008, Walshe 2003).

This is an extremely disturbing indictment of contemporary health and social care cultures and wider sociopolitical structures in the UK. However, there is a glimmer of hope. The Francis (2013) and Andrews (2014) reports have noted this recurring pattern of failure and have suggested a different, and – one hopes – more effective kind of cultural change, focused on the values they believe lie at the very heart of a culture of care. Both suggest that if the values of care (see Table 13.1) are inherent in the individual practitioner, at the point of entry into professional training (ensured through a values-based recruitment process) (Francis 2013), and a 'psychological contract' can be constructed and maintained between employee and employer in practice settings (Andrews 2014, p.3), then a shared vision of care can be co-created within the organisational milieu.

In essence, these reports promote the development of a living, breathing culture of care that embeds 'improved support for compassionate, caring and committed care' (Francis 2013, p.66) and a process of 'genuinely listening' and responding to others (Keogh 2013, p.2). To support this 'caring' ethos, the NHS has developed a *Constitution* (DH 2009) which articulates the values and beliefs that employees and organisations must now hold in order to provide health and social care services (see Table 13.3).

Table 13.3 The principles and values of the NHS Constitution

Principles include providing:	Values include evidencing and embodying the following:
A comprehensive service, available to all, irrespective of gender, race, disability, age, sexual orientation, religion or belief.	Respect and dignity for each person as an individual, including valuing their aspirations, commitments, priorities, needs, abilities and limits. Also listening to others, recognising one's own limitations and being honest.
Access based on clinical need, *not* the ability to pay. NHS services are free at point of delivery.	Commitment to gaining trust by striving for the best quality of care at all times including: in terms of safety, confidentiality, professional and managerial integrity, accountability, dependability and good communication. Feedback is welcomed and action taken and learned from.
A service that aspires to the highest standards of excellence and professionalism, including development and support of staff as well as care and treatment of patients.	Compassion for others, i.e. the ability to respond with humanity and kindness to each person's pain, distress, anxiety or need. Time is found for those we serve and work alongside and acts of kindness offered, however small.

A service that must reflect the needs and preferences of the patients, their families and their carers. Patients are valued partners, not passive recipients.	Improving lives by striving to improve health and well-being and people's experiences of the NHS.
A service that works across organisational boundaries and in partnership with others, in the interests of patients, local communities and the wider population.	Working together for patients by putting patients first in everything that is done and ensuring their needs are placed before organisational boundaries.
A service that is committed to best value (in terms of the use of taxpayers' money) and the most sustainable, effective and fair use of resources.	To ensure that everyone counts by using resources for the benefit of the patients and the whole community; accepting that, where resources are finite, difficult decisions do have to be made.
A service that is accountable to the public, the communities and patients that it serves. It takes decisions locally and facilitates scrutiny of its performance and priorities.	

Adapted from DH 2009.

The principles and values of the NHS *Constitution*

The NHS *Constitution* (DH 2009) identifies seven principles and six key values that, in theory at least, underpin the philosophy or the foundational beliefs of the whole system of health and social care in the United Kingdom. Specifically, these values and principles work together to define the ethical frameworks and beliefs that guide behaviour and decision-making processes in both the organisation and the individual practitioners who work in these settings (see Table 13.3).

The organisational context

The principles (i.e. the underpinning philosophy or foundational beliefs of the NHS *Constitution*) offer a shared framework of essential characteristics that define the nature and practice of the organisational context. In terms of health care in the UK, this means that:

- Access to services is based on need, *not* the ability to pay.
- Service users/patients receive high-quality, evidence-based care, at all times. Failings in this basic provision of care are prominent in the reports in Table 13.2.
- Services (organisations and their respective teams) must work in partnership with others across organisational boundaries (i.e. public, private and third sector agencies). The inability to do this was a significant failure in many of the reports noted in Table 13.2. It continues to be a challenge at the time of writing this chapter.

- Services (organisations and their respective teams) are accountable (or answerable) to those they serve. This was another commonly missing factor evidenced in the reports in Table 13.2.
- Performance is not only based on best value for money, but also on the values of care, reflecting the needs and preferences (or choices) of service users. In many, if not all, of the examples shared in the reports in Table 13.2, there was a clear tendency to prioritise 'best value' (in terms of financial savings), to the detriment of meeting service users' needs and preferences (in terms of care).

Reflective questions

- Why do you think money can so often be put before the needs of people (think about clients/patients and staff here), especially when history shows us what happens when this is done?
- What are the qualities you think a caring organisation should have?
- Have you experienced working in a caring environment? If so, what did it *look* like and how did it feel?

The person context

Whilst the *principles* of the NHS *Constitution* (see Table 13.3) can be observed and to some extent measured in practice, the accompanying *values* are, by their nature, more subjective and serve to guide how individual practitioners in the field should behave in any given situation. The NHS *Constitution* maintains that these values should be inherent qualities in all workers, both individually and collectively, because then, and only then, can these values be evidenced through our everyday behaviours and practice. Although this list is by no means complete, these behaviours will include:

- evidencing and practising respect and dignity toward others, at all times, irrespective of personal issues or the levels of stress and pressure in the workplace.
- a caring and compassionate approach in practice that strives to meet the needs of others, at all times, irrespective of personal issues or the levels of stress and pressure in the workplace.
- striving to improve health and well-being at all times, irrespective of personal issues or the levels of stress and pressure in the workplace.
- excellence in professionalism and everyday practice at all times, irrespective of personal issues or the levels of stress and pressure in the workplace
- putting the needs of patients and communities first, before organisational boundaries, irrespective of personal issues or the levels of stress and pressure in the workplace.

- using resources for the benefit of people and sharing that equitably, whilst recognising that difficult decisions might have to be made, irrespective of personal issues or the levels of stress and pressure in the workplace.
(Adapted from DH 2009).

On first reading this, it would seem like common sense that those who *choose* to work in the caring professions, or offer supporting roles in health and social care fields, would believe in these principles and values; you might be thinking, 'Well of course I would do that'. Sadly, as Table 13.2 attests, history has shown that organisational cultures have pushed staff to put concerns about saving money and meeting targets *before* caring for the vulnerable people they were supposed to protect and indeed before caring for themselves. This has resulted in high levels of burnout and stress in health and social care settings (Clouston 2014, 2015). So what can we do? This is our challenge and the challenge of the NHS *Constitution*. Working together, the integration of the Constitution's principles and values are now setting out the blueprint for a new caring culture that each and every worker and each and every organisation will have to embody. Again, this sounds great, but it is not easy to implement.

On a personal level, it might mean having to make changes in the way you behave, practise or interact; you might have to confront your own moral compass (your notions of right and wrong in terms of conduct: see Figure 13.1) and your way of thinking about certain people, behaviours or attitudes. You may have to challenge the organisation you work for or colleagues you work with, because they are not meeting the values and principles expected of a caring environment. On an organisational level, cultural change will not only have to happen in terms of beliefs, values and behaviours but in all cultural dimensions, including structure, systems, orientation, drives, identification and levels of acceptance (Hofstede *et al.* 1990). None of these changes are easy to make, but they are essential in order to create a culture of care. Moreover, they all have to be valued and maintained collectively if the overall change is to work.

Reflective questions

- Think about your personal values in terms of being caring; try to name the caring qualities you have. How do you evidence these values and qualities to others and in your everyday practice in the workplace?
- What do the words 'care' and 'compassion' mean to you? How would you define them and how would you reflect this in your practice?
- What do the words 'dignity' and 'respect' mean to you? How can you evidence this in your everyday practice?

- Consider Case study 13.1. Reflect on how you would do this differently if you were the staff member.

Case study 13.1 Care, compassion, dignity and respect

Enid was an 84-year-old woman who had been admitted to hospital with pneumonia. Prior to her admission to hospital, she was eating well and living independently in a three-bedroomed house. However, since admission, her condition had deteriorated and the family and care team had decided a care home or support package was necessary for safe discharge.

Enid was desperate to go home but the social worker had been unable to action the care package needed to support her and could not find a place in a care home, either temporarily or permanently.

As a result of her increasing hospital stay and bed rest, her feet had become swollen and ulcerated; she was experiencing difficulty in walking and transferring, but was still mobile with assistance. The nursing staff were keen to get her up and ambulating in order to reduce the swelling in her feet and relieve the pressure on the base of her spine, as there was evidence of early-stage skin breakdown.

It was visiting time on the ward and Enid had her son and daughter-in-law present. Enid told her daughter-in-law she needed to go to the toilet urgently, noting that she had been given a suppository earlier in the day because there had been some difficulties in passing motions. Her son went to find a nurse to help to take Enid to the toilet. He was gone over 10 minutes because he could not find a member of staff. He eventually located a nurse who said she would see what she could do.

About 5 minutes after returning to the ward, a health care support worker entered the seven-bedded bay with the tea trolley. From the doorway, she shouted across to Enid, 'I know you want to go the loo Enid, love. I'll just get you a commode and put the curtains round.'

Enid was distressed that her need to use the toilet had been announced to all present, but told her family she could not wait any longer; this was relayed privately to the support worker who brought the commode about 5 minutes later.

> However, by this time Enid had passed her motion and the support worker asked the visitors to leave in order to clean Enid and strip the bed. She chided Enid in front of the visitors and told her she was a naughty girl not to have asked sooner. It was now over 20 minutes since the initial request had been made.
>
> When the visitors were able to return, Enid was very distressed and crying, saying she was mortified. The family complained to the ward sister who said Enid's behaviour was 'difficult' and she was very demanding. She noted that the support worker had done what was necessary and suggested that Enid should have been timelier in her request for toileting as they were very busy and it took time to action support.

Why are values important?

Piglet sidled up to Pooh from behind.

'Pooh!' he whispered.

'Yes Piglet?'

'Nothing,' said Piglet, taking Pooh's paw. 'I just wanted to be sure of you.'

(Milne 1994, p.209)

To recap, values are important because they reflect and shape our social norms, and wider cultural beliefs; they also shape our ethical framework and behaviours. Subsequently, they influence organisational and personal behaviours, affecting how we, individually and in groups, behave in our everyday lives. Values incorporate social and cultural principles (social norms, if you like) but also interpersonal skills (how we interact with others); in this way, they shape the individual's beliefs and the ethical or moral compass we use to understand the world we live in and make personal judgements and decisions.

When values are understood in this multifaceted way, their importance in the health and social arena becomes clear: if values are inherent aspects of who we are and how we think and feel, they are pivotal to how we behave. Consequently, values influence and frame the choices we make and the attitudes we hold toward others, not only in our everyday lives but also in our work. In the context of care and professional practice, it is crucial to understand this because we all use values to make decisions every day. Values are therefore central to, and reflected in, the choices we make, our judgements, and thus our ethical decision-making in our personal and professional or work-based lives. (Think, for example, about how you would have done things differently in Case study 13.1.)

As health and social care workers, we learn about values in our education or professional subject pedagogy (specific methods or practices used to teach a certain subject). However, because we are also unique individuals, our personal values and beliefs, our ethical lens or moral compass, will also influence what we do and the choices we make. This is why individual differences exist and why values-based recruitment has been promoted: if we each interpret wider contextual values or principles differently because we have a unique lens, then it is important to ensure that our moral compass is pointing in the right direction before we begin our professional training. Would Harold Shipman and Beverley Allitt (see Table 13.2) have been accepted into medicine and nursing respectively had values-based recruitment been in place? One would hope not.

So, what might the core or essential values of a candidate for health and social care work look like? An ideal moral compass is shown in Figure 13.1. Remember this is not exclusive and may vary somewhat from person to person. Look at this along with the definitions and associated behaviours listed in Table 13.1.

Note the ability to be reflective and to have the ability to grow and change in Figure 13.1. These are essential qualities for any health and social care worker and they are integral to the ethics and standards of practice. Think about these qualities in relation to your own profession and personal practice and ensure you can articulate why reflection and the ability to challenge your own thinking are important. Note also the 'transcendent lens' mentioned in the top middle quality. We will return to both these points later.

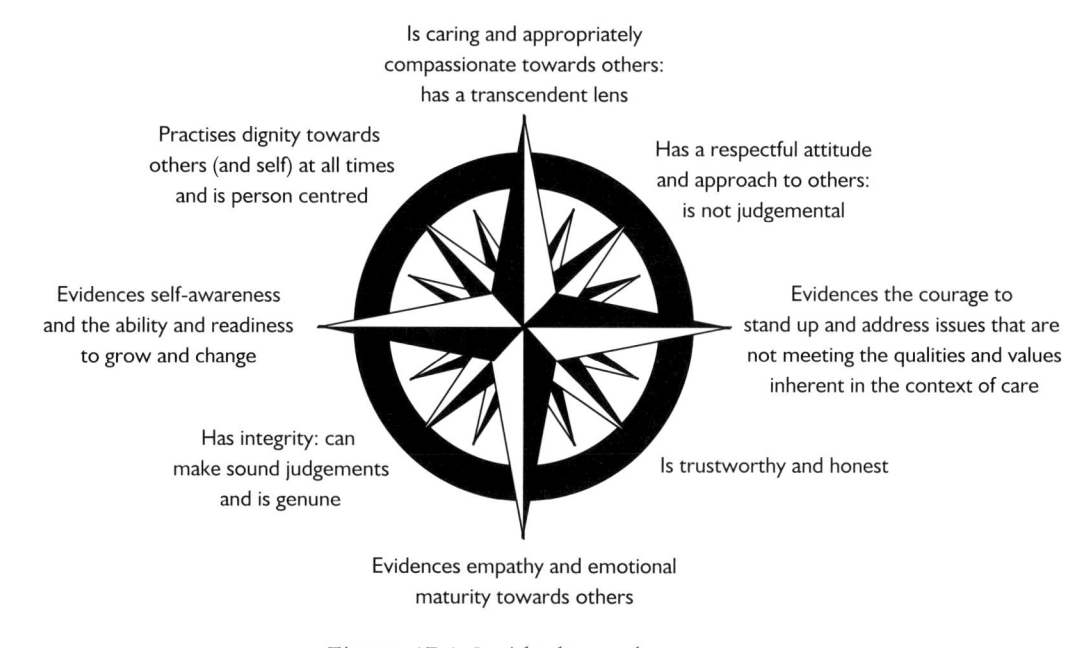

Figure 13.1 An ideal moral compass

Reflective questions

- Reflect on and plot what your own moral compass might look like. Then look at Figure 13.1 and compare and contrast it with your own.
- On reflection, do you feel you would like to work on some aspect of your own moral compass and develop or address a particular value further?
- Can you think of a situation where your moral compass differed from somebody else's? What were the moral and ethical values that underpinned these differences?
- Would you expand on or adapt the compass in Figure 13.1 for health and social care workers? If so, how would you do this and why?

Making the right choices

If values are the inherent beliefs that shape our collective behaviour as well as shaping our individual characters, and we all behave differently because we each have a unique ethical lens or moral compass, how can we learn to make different choices when we make decisions? In other words, how can we change and adapt our personal moral compass? And how can we adjust the way we act towards others in order to meet their individual needs? According to Argandona (2003), this is possible because we all evaluate the potential outcomes of any choices or decisions we make, using three criteria, or lenses:

- **The personal or intrinsic lens**: When utilising this lens, we ask ourselves, 'What will the imagined outcome of this decision mean for me, personally?'
- **The extrinsic or organisational and/or professional lens**: When utilising this lens, we ask ourselves, 'What will the imagined outcome of this decision mean for me, in terms of expectations in my workplace, my career aspirations or social/cultural capital?'
- **The transcendent or significant other lens**: When utilising this lens, we ask ourselves, 'What will the imagined outcome of this decision mean for others?' These 'others' will include our patient/clients but also our family, colleagues, workmates or additional significant others.

These three lenses are very important because they allow us to see how we can apply a more personally individualised 'me' lens or a professional and/or organisationally constructed 'outcome' lens over a more person-centred patient/client 'impact on others' lens. Some possible outcomes of *not* applying the transcendent lens are described in the reports noted in Table 13.2. This is not to say that all lenses do not have necessary elements that we might have to consider at any one time and in any particular decision-making situation; but in a health and social care context, it is about adjusting these lenses so they are more appropriately focused to meet the needs of the patient/client first and other stakeholders (like you and the organisation) second.

How can you adjust your lens?

The simple truth is that you have to accept that there is a need to think before you act and essentially to start to put others, specifically patients and clients, before your own personal gain and before organisational drivers, if they are at odds with 'being caring'. Professional standards, of course, shape the way we do things every day, and we can lose our jobs and careers if we do not follow them. However, it is worth reflecting on how your professional lens could benefit from a more person-centred, caring approach and whether bureaucracy or interpretation in some organisational settings has perhaps misinterpreted the essence of professional practice; these factors certainly played some part in the errors in judgement and decision-making that reports like Francis (2013) and Andrews (2014) identified.

It is not easy to adjust your thinking and perspectives to put others before yourself, especially when the organisation might be driving you to work longer and harder, and to meet specific performance outcomes, but it is essential if we are to create a caring transcendent culture to promote real and meaningful change.

What might get in the way of making transcendent change?

As mentioned previously, this kind of cultural change is not easy. On a personal level, challenging how you personally think and behave is a reflective process; it is a form of *transformational* or deep personal learning (Mezirow 1997). It is this depth that causes you to critically consider the reality of the situation and the options available to you – and thus enables you to reflect and adjust your moral compass, your decision-making processes and your interpersonal skills.

However, individual change is not enough: for cultural change to work at a values-based level, those values have to be shared. In the context of health and social care, this means a collective approach by all members of an organisation to caring, compassion, dignity and respect, as well as all the other values noted in Table 13.1.

To date, as the reports in Table 13.2 verify, this shared value base has not been achieved; mistakes have occurred and when people have challenged organisational cultures or raised concerns about the behaviour of colleagues, they have been treated badly, bullied or constructively dismissed (Francis 2013). Whistleblowing (disclosing or raising concerns over wrongdoing, malpractice or uncaring or unethical behaviours, values or attitudes in the workplace) wrongly took on negative connotations, but this is being pragmatically addressed. Raising and escalating concerns is now a necessary, and indeed required, professional skill (HCPCl 2016, standard 7). This is supported by the need to be open and honest when things go wrong, and gaining the ability to reflect on your own part in any one situation and address it (HCPC 2016, standard 8). But what else needs to be done to ensure that this values-based culture becomes normative?

People, professions and organisations

According to Fry *et al.* (2012, p. 208), 'When moral sensibility (values, beliefs and morals) are challenged, negative emotions such as dissatisfaction and frustration are experienced.' However, the problem with having an individual, professional and organisationally shared value system is that value congruence (match) between these different stakeholders can be challenging (Fitzgerald & Desjardins 2004). For values to become normative at all levels, they need to be clearly defined and communicated by the organisation so they can become a shared way of being for all members.

This idea of the sharing of values is the basis of the psychological contract that appears in the recommendations of the Andrews report (see Table 13.2). A psychological contract requires all members of the organisation to share a common values system, at an emotional and psychological level. This should be very easy to achieve in health and social care settings: individual practitioners and professional groups working in these fields all adhere to standards and ethical frameworks that promote such values, forming a common thread that can bind them together.

However, the definitions of these values need to be clarified. Behaviours need to be identified and reinforced to enable meaningful change to be made and become a continual process; without these clear parameters, full consciousness and attention to caring can lapse. This is particularly important when new values are being adopted because it requires ongoing investment from the organisation and its stakeholders (in this case the UK government and the public who fund and use the services) to make it work. It is therefore important to consider how the underlying market forces that affect funding for health and social care can impact on the agendas of organisations and their stakeholders, and how these, in turn, can influence caring values.

You will recall that the common failure among all the inquiries noted in Table 13.2 (and many others not mentioned) was the particular organisation's drive to meet financially driven government and organisational outcomes rather than caring value (see Francis 2013 for evidence).

Market forces and health care

Illiffe (2008, p. 3) comments that 'Medicine is changing from a craft concerned with the uniqueness of each encounter with an ill person to a mass-manufacturing industry preoccupied with the throughput of the sick.' It is true that market forces have played a major part in UK government policy since the Thatcher government of the 1980s. According to the political philosophy known as neoliberalism, market forces drive consumerism, productivity and growth. They also provide the basis for privatisation of public services (such as health and social care) and promote individual responsibility over shared, collective accountability.

At first glance, this may not seem problematic: financial growth and productivity apparently create stability and security; and placing responsibility with the individual means they are personally accountable when things go wrong. However, for health and social care services in the UK, the impact of this philosophy has been far-reaching: there is a lack of investment from government in these services, resulting in fewer resources. This increases the pressure on staff to do more with less, and increases the stress and responsibilities placed on individual workers (Clouston 2014, 2015). As the reports in Table 13.2 attest, it is these very factors that have promoted the growth of the organisational lens as a predominant perspective in health and social care, and consequently caused many of the reported failings by increasing pressures and creating ethical tensions and dilemmas for staff (Kinsella & Pittman 2012).

Reflective questions

- Can you think of a situation where you made a personally orientated decision when it should or could have been more transcendent? If so, what would you do differently now, and how would the outcome be different?
- Can you think of a situation where you made an organisationally orientated decision when it should or could have been more transcendent? If so, what would you do differently now and how would the outcome be different?
- Consider how you could realise the transcendent outcome. In other words, consider the impact on the patient/client or – more generally – the 'other', into your everyday decision-making scenarios.

Engendering care and compassion in health and social care

> We respond with humanity and kindness to each person's pain, distress, anxiety or need. We search for the things we can do, however small, to give comfort and relieve suffering. We find time for those we serve and work alongside. We do not wait to be asked, because we care.
>
> NHS Constitution *(DH 2009, p.26)*

To summarise, health and social care professionals are all expected to be inherently caring in their philosophy and hold this value as a basic and profound belief. Showing empathy and compassion and treating others with dignity and respect are behaviours that demonstrate caring in the everyday practice setting (Doyle et al. 2014, Firth-Cozens & Cornwell 2009).

Nevertheless, these behaviours can seem a little vague. For instance, how do you actually demonstrate empathy and compassion? It is perhaps harder to articulate what such behaviours *should* look like than what they should not look like. Moreover, as we have discussed, and Francis (2013), Andrews (2014) as well as other reports have all evidenced, it can be challenging to practise care and compassion in a setting where you feel pressured by time constraints and limited staff resources, because these promote achieving performance outcomes.

Common sense would suggest that, with a little forethought, and an assurance that our moral compass is pointing in the right direction, we, as human beings, can and do make sound judgements and decisions all the time. However, values are tacit and it is therefore helpful to have a common understanding of what we mean by these values and their associated behaviours.

You will recall that Table 13.1 (p. 166) gave an overview of common definitions and examples of 'caring' behaviours. To support your understanding further, there are a couple of models in health and social care literature that may help you to consider some of these values and skills in a more practical and profession-specific way.

However, these models are by no means a panacea and, when you read about them, you do need to use a critical and transcendent lens. Each one has its roots in a different professional group – and thus subject pedagogy. For example, Epstein and Hundert's (2002) 'Professional Competence Model' emerged from the medical model of care and has a rather practical approach to caring values, based around competence and skill. This model could certainly be built on further in the present climate.

The 'Intentional Relationship Model' was developed by occupational therapists and theoretically promotes a more psychosocial perspective (Taylor 2008), focusing on the deliberate use of self as a therapeutic tool. Its basic premise is that practitioners can learn to adopt different *modes* or *interpersonal styles* with different clients/ patients, depending on that person's unique needs; so, in essence, you adapt yourself to the other. You could say this approach was very person-centred, but do look at the wording of the model and consider it with a critical and transcendent lens. Ask yourself, could it be improved upon? And if so, how? For example, could it be more driven by the client/patient?

Finally, the now well-known '6 Cs Model' was originally developed by nurses for nurses, specifically to engender caring and compassionate practice following the Francis inquiry (2013). It is the most recent of these values-based models and it appears to be, at least in terms of its lexicon, the most directly focused on caring values. Indeed, because it was specifically developed to address caring values, it has now been rolled out as a blueprint for all health and social care workers in the UK and thus, at least in theory, can be used as a guide to caring values along with the other models and the NHS Constitution. However, although promoted as ideal practice, again, do look at this model with a critical and transcendent lens. I would suggest there are many ways in which its discourse, meanings and actions (in terms of behaviour and outcome) could be improved to encapsulate meaningful compassionate care.

Table 13.4 summarises the key elements of all three of these models and gives you an opportunity to consider the similarities and differences between them, to think about how you might improve them and to enact caring values in different practice situations. But look carefully at their use of words and the meanings these convey, as I, for one, am not convinced they actually challenge the core of caring values as effectively as they could.

Table 13.4 Three models of care

7 Dimensions of Professional Competence (adapted from Epstein & Hundert 2002)	
Cognitive	Core knowledge, basic communication skills, information management, applying real world solutions, using tacit knowledge and personal experience, abstract problem-solving; self-directed acquisition of new knowledge; recognising gaps in knowledge, generating questions, using resources, e.g. evidence-based practice (EBP), research colleagues and learning from experience.
Technical	Competence in practical skills, e.g. physical exam, procedures, surgical skills. This is about competence in knowledge and skills.
Integrative	Incorporating scientific clinical and humanistic judgement; using clinical reasoning skills appropriately (e.g. hypothetico-deductive, pattern recognition, elaborated knowledge). Linking knowledge across disciplines and managing uncertainty.
Context	Applying skills competently in the clinical setting, appropriate to the specific client and use of time in the setting.
Relationship	Communication skills, handling conflict, teamwork, teaching others (e.g. patients, students and colleagues).
Affective/ moral	Tolerance of ambiguity and anxiety, emotional intelligence, respect for patients, responsiveness to patients and society, being caring.
Habits of mind	Observations of one's own thinking, emotions, techniques, attentiveness, critical curiosity, recognition of and response to cognitive and emotional biases; willingness to recognise and correct errors, i.e. to change and grow.

7 Modes of Practice (adapted from Taylor et al. 2009, original 6 modes)	
Problem-solving	Facilitating pragmatic thinking, and solving dilemmas by outlining choices (informed choices), posing questions and providing opportunities for comparative or analytical thinking.
Instructing	Structuring therapy activities and being explicit with the client/s about the plan, sequence and events of therapy. Providing clear instructions and feedback about performance; setting limits on the client's requests and behaviour.
Encouraging	Striving to provide the client with confidence, hope, courage, and the will to explore or perform a given activity (therapy/ treatment).
Advocating	Ensuring the client's rights are enforced and resources secured. Acting as mediator, facilitator, negotiator, enforcer or otherwise to respond to physical, social, and environmental barriers that the client encounters.
Collaborating	Expecting the client to be an active and equal participant in therapy; ensuring choice, freedom and autonomy to the greatest possible extent; getting feedback from the client before choosing or recommending any activity; asking a client to recommend their own goals for therapy.
Empathising	Bearing witness to and striving to fully understand the client's physical, psychological, interpersonal and emotional experience. Ensuring the client verifies and validates the therapist's understanding.
Reflective practice	This is a 7th mode added by Morrison (2013), who suggests that the ability to reflect is essential to the therapeutic relationship but maintains that this has to be balanced with an ability to recognise that environmental factors can be outside the therapist's control and that recognition of this is essential in terms of personal and professional resilience and well-being. This is a notable point and links to the notion of critical learning opportunities and the ability to transform or change personal perspectives and ways of being, in terms of professional practice (Clouston 2017).

6 Cs (adapted from DOH 2012b)	
Care	Care is the core business of individuals and organisations; it defines the nature of work and it helps to improve individual and community health.
Competence	Means all those in caring roles have to be able to understand the health and social needs of others and have the expertise, and clinical and technical knowledge to deliver effective care.
Courage	To do the right thing; speak up and challenge when there are concerns and to have the strength to innovate and embrace new ways of working.
Commitment	To patients and populations, a cornerstone of delivery; to build on the commitment to improve the care and experience of patients, to take action to make this vision and strategy a reality for all and meet the health, care and support challenges ahead.

Communication	Communication is central to successful caring relationships and to effective team working.
	Listening is as important as what we say and do and essential for 'no decision about me without me'. Communication is the key to a good workplace, with benefits for patients and staff alike.
Compassion	How care is given through relationships based on empathy, respect and dignity – it can also be described as intelligent kindness, and is central to how people perceive their care.

As a final reflective point for this chapter, allow yourself to fully absorb the meanings these models convey in terms of challenging values and changing behaviour and ask yourself what is missing? The missing factors are often the critical elements we can learn so much from; and bringing these factors into the light often enables us to facilitate the most meaningful learning and thus transformational change.

Conclusion

So, what have you learned on your journey through this chapter? In reality, this is for you to decide; but we hope you have come to understand that the caring values in health and social care practice are about being reflexive and open to change, challenging your own thinking, coming to know and, if necessary, adapting your own moral compass, putting patients/clients (and other people) first, and meeting their needs before organisational and personal requirements at all times. Whilst this is imperative to caring, it is also about having the courage and integrity to challenge values and behaviours that do not reflect these principles and values and advocating for those who lack the power or ability to do so for themselves.

Adopting these values and being caring and compassionate is not necessarily easy, but it is rewarding; it is about valuing others as a part of being authentically you. As a caring professional, these are critical qualities, requiring wisdom, courage and humility along with the ability to hold and develop a transcendent lens with integrity. It is a worthy and meaningful journey filled with the pleasure of genuinely and warmly caring for others; there is no greater gift to give than this.

References

Andrews Report. (2014). *Trusted to Care: An Independent Review of the Princess of Wales Hospital and Neath Port Talbot Hospital at ABMU Health Board.* Cardiff: Dementia Services Development Centre.

Argandona, A. (2003). Fostering values in organizations. *Journal of Business Ethics*. **45**, 15–28.

Calnan, M. & Rowe, R. (2004). *Trust in Health Care: An Agenda for Future Research.* London: Nuffield Trust.

Clothier Report (1994). *Independent Inquiry Relating to Deaths and Injuries on the Children's Wards at Grantham and Kesteven Hospital.* London: The Stationery Office.

Clouston, T.J. (2014). Whose occupational balance is it anyway? The challenge of neoliberal capitalism and work-life imbalance. *British Journal of Occupational Therapy.* **77** (10), 507–15.

Clouston, T.J. (2015). *Challenging Stress, Burnout and Rust-out: Finding Balance in Busy Lives.* London: Jessica Kingsley.

Clouston, T.J. (2017). Transforming learning: teaching compassion and caring values in higher education. *Journal of Further and Higher Education.* http://dx.doi.org/10.1080/0309877X.2017.1332359 (last accessed 24.11.2017)

Coulter, A., and Collins, A. (2011). *Making Shared Decision-Making a Reality: No Decision About Me, Without Me.* London: King's Fund.

Department of Health (DH) (2009). *The NHS Constitution.* London: DH.

Department of Health (DH) (2012a). *Transforming Care: A National Response to Winterbourne View Hospital.* London: DH.

Department of Health (DH) (2012b). *Compassion in Practice: Nursing Midwifery and Care Staff our Vision and Strategy.* London: DH.

Doyle, K., Hungerford, C. & Cruickshank, M. (2014). Reviewing tribunal cases and nurse behaviour: Putting empathy back into nurse education with Bloom's taxonomy. *Nurse Education Today.* **34** (7), 1069–73.

Epstein, R. & Hundert, E. (2002). Defining and assessing professional competence. *Journal of the American Medical Association (JAMA).* **287** (2), 226–35.

Firth-Cozens, J. & Cornwell, J. (2009). *The Point of Care: Enabling Compassionate Care in Acute Hospital Settings.* London: King's Fund.

Fitzgerald, G.A. & Desjardins, N.M. (2004). Organizational values and their relation to organizational performance outcomes. *Atlantic Journal of Communication.* **12** (3), 121–45.

Francis, R. (2013). *Report of the Mid Staffordshire NHS Foundation Trust Public Inquiry.* London: The Stationery Office.

Fry, M., Ruperto, K., Jarrett, K., Wheeler, J., Fong, J. & Fetchett, W. (2012). Managing the wait: clinical initiative nurses' perceptions of an extended scope practice role. *Australasian Emergency Nursing Journal.* **15** (4), 202–210.

Galloway, J. (2013). *Dignity, values, attitudes and person-centred care.* https://www.esht.nhs.uk/wp-content/uploads/2017/08/Dignity-values-attitudes-and-person-centred-care.pdf (last accessed 18.09.2017)

Halpern, J. (2003). What is clinical empathy? *Journal of General Internal Medicine.* **18**, 670–74.

Hardee, J.T. (2003). Health systems: An overview of empathy. *The Permanente Journal.* **7** (4), 51–53.

Haringey Serious Case Review (2009). Haringey, London: Local Safeguarding Children Board.

Health and Care Professions Council (HCPC) (2016). *Standards of conduct, performance and ethics.* London: HCPC.

Hofstede, G., Neuijen, B., Ohayv, D. & Sanders, G. (1990). Measuring organizational cultures: A qualitative and quantitative study across twenty cases. *Administrative Science Quarterly.* **35** (2) 286–316.

Iliffe, S. (2008). *From General Practice to Primary Care: The Industrialisation of Family Medicine.* Oxford: Oxford University Press.

Keogh, B. (2013). *Review into the Quality of Care and Treatment Provided by 14 Hospital Trusts in England: Overview Report.* London: NHS England.

Kinsella, E.A. & Pittman, A. (2012). *Phronesis as Professional Knowledge: Practical Wisdom in the Professionals.* Rotterdam: Sense Publishers.

Laming Report (2003). *The Climbié Inquiry. CM 5730.* London: The Stationery Office.

Laming Report (2009). *The Protection of Children in England: A Progress Report.* London: The Stationery Office.

Maslow, A. (1948). 'Higher' and 'Lower' Needs. *Journal of Psychology.* **25**, 433–36.

Mezirow, J. (1997). 'Transformative learning: Theory to practice' in P. Cranton (ed.) *Transformative Learning in Action: Insights from Practice. New Directions for Adult and Continuing Education: No. 74.* San Francisco, CA: Jossey-Bass.5–12.

Milne, A.A. (1994). *Winnie the Pooh: The Complete Collection of Stories and Poems.* London: Methuen.

Morrison, T.L. (2013). Individual and environmental implications of working alliances in Occupational Therapy. *British Journal of Occupational Therapy.* **76** (11), 507–514.

Paton, R.A. & McCalman, J. (2008). *Change Management: A Guide to Effective Implementation.* 3rd edn. Los Angeles: Sage Publications.

Phillips, A. & Taylor, B. (2009). *On Kindness.* London: Hamish Hamilton.

Platt, F.W. (1992). Empathy: can it be taught? *Annals Internal Medicine.* **117** (8), 700–701.

Public Interest Disclosure Act (1998). http://www.legislation.gov.uk/ukpga/1998/23/contents (last accessed 13.09.2017).

Shipman Inquiry (2002). *Death Disguised.* London: The Stationery Office.

Shipman Inquiry (2003a). *The Police Investigation of March 1998.* London: The Stationery Office.

Shipman Inquiry (2003b). *Death Certification and the Investigation of Deaths by Coroners.* London: The Stationery Office.

Shipman Inquiry (2004a). *The Regulation of Controlled Drugs in the Community.* London: The Stationery Office.

Shipman Inquiry (2004b). *Safeguarding Patients: Lessons from the Past – Proposals for the Future.* London: The Stationery Office.

Shipman Inquiry (2005). *Shipman: the Final Report.* London: The Stationery Office.

Sinclair, S., Norris, J.M., McConnell, S.J., Chochinov, H.M., Hack, T.F., Hagen, N.A., McClement, S. & Bouchal, S.R. (2016). Compassion: a scoping review of the healthcare literature. *BMC Palliative Care.* **15** (6), 1–16.

Solmon, B. & Clouston, T.J. (2016). Occupational therapy and the therapeutic use of self. *British Journal of Occupational Therapy.* **79** (8), 514–516.

Taylor, R.R. (2008). *The Intentional Relationship: Occupational Therapy and Use of Self.* Philadelphia: F.A. Davis Company.

Taylor, R.R., Lee, W.S., Kielhofner, G. & Ketkar, M. (2009). Therapeutic use of self: A nationwide survey of practitioners' attitudes and experiences. *American Journal of Occupational Therapy.* **63** (2), 198–207.

Walshe, K. (2003). *Inquiries: Learning from Failure in the NHS.* London: The Nuffield Trust.

Watterson, L. (2013). 6Cs + Principles = Care. *Nursing Standard.* **27** (46), 24–25.

Winterbourne View: Time for change (2014). London: NHS England.

Chapter 14

The place of spirituality in health and social care practice

Melody Cranbourne-Rosser

Learning outcomes

By the end of this chapter you will be able to:

- Understand the essence of spirituality and why it is important in health and social care practice
- Consider how spirituality can inform and influence care and caring values within a variety of contexts
- Appreciate the relevance of spirituality for service users and for practitioner care and well-being in the healing context
- Identify and reflect upon your own concepts of spirituality and how they may need to be adapted or considered in your everyday practice and attitudes to others.

What is spirituality and why is it important?

Spirituality holds a significant position in the lives of many and therefore requires an equally significant response from those working within health and social care. Research and clinical experience highlight the complexity of this topic and suggest that spiritual beliefs and practices can be largely beneficial but also harmful in certain circumstances. For example, certain beliefs and practices can promote resilience and recovery (Royal College of Psychiatrists 2011), help sustain those living with long-term illness or nearing the end of life (Candy *et al.* 2009), bring a sense of meaning to challenging experiences (Gilbert & Parkes 2011), and provide a unique perspective when assessing and enhancing quality of life (O'Connell & Skevington 2010).

However, spiritual beliefs can also have the potential to exacerbate or trigger mental health problems (Koenig *et al.* 2012); and are used by some to control or harm others (Orlowski 2010, Jenkinson 2013, Oakley & Kinmond 2013). If we neglect the spiritual dimension of human experience, we risk failing to deliver a truly holistic framework of care; this in turn can lead to the risk of missing both the health-promoting and health-diminishing effects of related beliefs, practices and experiences.

Grasping sand: defining spirituality

Spirituality is a difficult concept to define, partly due to its subtle and somewhat enigmatic nature, but also because of the richly diverse forms it takes, and our tendency to use certain terms, such as 'religion' and 'spirituality', interchangeably. For some, spirituality relates to a particular religious system that helps people frame their understanding of the world. For others, it may hold a very different meaning, as they do not identify with any particular organised religious groups or practices. For example, those who consider themselves 'spiritual but not religious' may speak of perceiving the depth, magic and mystery of the natural world and possibly an 'intelligence' behind its unfolding patterns; or they may speak in terms of a sense of connection to self, others, nature, or the wider cosmos. Some may not consider spirituality to have any role in their lives. All such viewpoints are equally valid and are an important part of who we are. Before going any further, I would like to invite you to reflect on material covered in this chapter from a personal perspective by considering the following questions.

Reflective questions

- What does the term 'spirituality' mean to me?
- Would I consider myself to have a spiritual life?
- If yes, how do I experience and express this on a day-to-day basis?
- If not, how do I feel about being asked to consider it?

Researchers and clinicians alike have attempted to develop definitions that somehow capture spirituality and its multifaceted makeup, even though condensing this complex concept into a single paragraph does not do it justice. However, a definition may offer a helpful starting point, even though it is likely to be far from complete. With this in mind I would like to share a description proposed by Swinton (2001, p.20):

> Spirituality is … an intra, inter and transpersonal experience that is shaped and directed by the experiences of individuals and of the communities within which they live out their lives. It is intrapersonal in that it refers to the quest for inner connectivity … interpersonal in that it relates to the relationship between people and within communities … [and] transpersonal in so far as it reaches beyond self and others into the transcendent realms of experience that move beyond that which is available at a mundane level.

I would also like to highlight some key themes identified by Gilbert and Parkes (2011, p.2), who noted that spirituality provided 'meaning, purpose and a sense of grounding', was a 'source of hope, values, and worth', related to 'anything from which a person derives purpose, hope and self-acceptance', and involved 'connecting with self, others, and "other" (has a transcendent element)'.

For ease of writing I will use the word 'spirituality' to refer to all possible ways of experiencing and expressing that which might fall under this label. Although this word may make some feel uncomfortable, I would ask that you put aside, where possible, any tension this may bring, and simply superimpose any word or term that better suits your unique perspective, while at the same time consider how those utilising health and social care services may hold similar or differing views.

Soul care

'Soul', a word that is commonly used alongside the term 'spirituality', is another of those 'S' words that requires consideration and negotiation. While listening to clients and colleagues alike, I have, on many occasions, heard them speak of what their soul 'needs' or may be 'trying to tell them' … if only they would sit still long enough to hear. Discussions regarding the soul abound throughout the realms of philosophy, neuroscience and psychology, to name but a few. What might the soul be? What is its nature? Does it exist at all? Debating such issues is beyond the scope of this chapter. However, what I would like to capture, at least in part, is the essence of how 'some' perceive the soul and briefly consider its place within the work we do with others.

Thomas Moore, in *Care of the Soul* (1998, p.23), acknowledged the soul to be the 'sense of the sacredness of each individual life … the unfathomable mystery that is the very seed and heart'. What we sense to be sacred within our inner and outer world will be particular to us and those we support. What is important here is that we somehow find a way to allow space for that which is 'sacred' within the lives of others – the essential aspect that provides meaning and purpose. If we fail to allow space for this, we fail to acknowledge a person's deepest sense of self and place within the world – or, by shifting the focus briefly back to ourselves, that which brings meaning and purpose to our own existence, whether it relates to work, personal interests, relationships, or connectedness to the deeper aspects of our inner life.

Reflective questions

- Do I feel that I have (or am) a soul?
- If so, how do I know this? If not, how do I know this?
- How and when have those around me spoken of the soul and how did I respond?

Spirituality: central theme or merely an adjunct?

Although spirituality, in some capacity, can often be found in legislation and professional guidelines, there is a tendency for it to be treated as an adjunct. Clarke (2013, p.28), who considers spirituality in terms of nursing care, notes that, "due to staff working under an already intolerable burden of responsibility, spirituality has become a marginalised aspect of care. It may have become more embedded in nursing rhetoric, but it has not become embedded in nursing practice". The same might be said for professions such as social work (Holloway & Moss 2010), psychotherapy (Vieten & Scammell 2015), psychology (Culliford 2011) and psychiatry (Koenig 2013).

However, developments of late suggest that spirituality has gained a higher profile. Such developments do not come without their fair share of both controversy and support, but each encourages a debate as to how and why spirituality needs to be included in health and social care settings. For example, religious and spiritual problems have been included as a category within the *Diagnostic and Statistical Manual of Mental Disorders* (DSM-IV), accompanied by a warning against pathologising spiritual experiences that do not require a clinical response (Lukoff *et al.* 2011). Other developments include the formation of the Spirituality and Psychiatry Special Interest Group within the Royal College of Psychiatrists, BACP Spirituality (one of seven divisions within the British Association for Counselling and Psychotherapy), the Spirituality Special Interest Group within the Division of Counselling Psychology of the British Psychological Society, the publication of legislation such as *Standards for Spiritual Care in the NHS in Wales* (Welsh Government 2010), and numerous international conferences relating to spirituality within health and social care.

However, some have argued that oversight continues with regard to including spirituality within legislation; the Nursing and Midwifery Council's new code of conduct, for example, came into effect in March 2015 and failed to overtly mention spirituality, despite such references appearing in earlier drafts (McSherry & Ross 2015). A paucity of relevant information in terms of working with children has also been noted, along with a call to broaden the spectrum and to embed spirituality in practice in a fuller, more holistic way, rather than as an 'add-on' (Murphy *et al.* 2015). The debate is therefore likely to continue.

Reflective questions

- With regard to my work or education-related environment, in what ways and how well has spirituality been included?
- What difference, if any, has this made to me personally?
- How might this inform or influence the work I do with others?

Spirituality in context
Spirituality, mental health and transformational crisis

Research suggests that there is a positive correlation between mental health, spirituality and recovery (Lukoff *et al.* 1993, Rohricht *et al.* 2009, Koenig *et al.* 2012) and there has been growing interest in this phenomenon over recent years. In a review of the wider literature, Gilbert and Parkes (2011, p.9) found that over 75% of studies noted that spirituality plays a positive role in 'well-being, recovery and resilience'. Findings such as these have led to recommendations to embrace spiritual practices and beliefs when formulating and implementing care packages.

On the other hand, some studies have noted that spirituality can also be associated with the potential for mental health distress and other difficulties – for example, when negative feelings and low self-worth have been promoted as part of spiritual teachings (Gilbert & Parkes 2011). Concerns have also been raised about the risks of considering oneself spiritual but having no religious framework with which to accommodate experiences, sometimes resulting in a poorer sense of well-being (King *et al.* 2013).

As spirituality has the potential to help as well as hinder well-being, the importance of keeping both sides in mind seems evident. However, individual spiritual needs within health and social care are often ignored, pathologised and, at times, even ridiculed.

Reflective questions

- Have I witnessed someone being dismissed, made fun of, or promptly pathologically labelled without a full assessment of their needs due to them speaking of their spiritual beliefs and experiences?
- Have I (even if unintentionally) treated someone in this way?
- What impact may this have had on the person and the support they received?

Even though holistic, person-centred care is constantly promoted in the health and social care system, some staff may still be biased towards conventional approaches to spirituality, and this may add to the problems experienced by some patients/service users. One such example is taken from the Department of Health (2011, p.62), who noted that:

> People who hold religious or other beliefs … have poorer experiences of services because core aspects of their identity are overlooked … [which] may cause anxiety and prove detrimental to their recovery.

Such concerns continue even though it is now recognised that spiritual beliefs and practices 'may be protective, particularly in relation to suicide' (Department of Health 2011, p.62). Appeals have been made by health professionals, carers and service users alike for spirituality to be more readily embraced and included in health and social care services, in line with a 'broader movement towards dignity, empowerment, personalisation, cultural identity and recovery' (Gilbert & Parkes 2011, p.14). For many, spirituality is an important part of their personal journey. Therefore, for a whole-person response to be offered, it needs to be respectfully and appropriately included in the overall package of care.

In addition to acknowledging the connection between spirituality and mental health, it has been proposed that, for some, the manifestation of certain signs and symptoms may not necessitate a clinical response, or perhaps not 'only' a clinical response if an individual would benefit from both this and another form of support. In other words, an individual's difficulties may be due to a transformative (or spiritual) crisis, rather than a purely mental health concern, and they may present with a range of intense and unexpected experiences, such as non-ordinary states of consciousness, overwhelming emotions, unusual physical manifestations, and thoughts and sensations that have mystical or religious themes running through them. An individual may also be faced with a complete overturning of their beliefs and sense of meaning due to loss, trauma and other challenging life experiences, leading to what might be considered a spiritual crisis.

Such experiences can be very complex and may lead to varying levels of disorientation, distress and disruption, as well as uncovering new insights and deeper understanding. The individual may be able to manage these experiences without external input, or they may require or benefit from support from their wider personal network and/or health and social care professionals who are open to the deep spiritual dimensions of the human experience.

Differentiating between a spiritual crisis (sometimes known as a spiritual emergency) and pathological experiences can be challenging. We need to consider the person's coping mechanisms and beliefs as well as their social and cultural background. Research continues to be undertaken to assist professionals in this task (Kaminker & Lukoff 2013), and, although there are still limitations with regard to differentiating between psychosis and spiritually transformative experiences, material is available that can act, at least in part, as a guide (Brett 2010). For example, a repository of related articles, leaflets and professional guidelines, written by members of the Spirituality and Psychiatry Special Interest Group, can be found on the website of the Royal College of Psychiatrists. Other resources can be accessed from the Spiritual Crisis Network and Spiritual Competency Resource Centre.

For the purposes of this chapter, it should be remembered that manifestations of mental ill-health may be the result of many factors, including transformational experiences which may need a different or broader response, as well as a respectful appreciation of the spiritual life of the individual involved. When researching transformative crisis, Brett (2010, p.173) identified an 'attitude of *learning from experience*'. This refers to the fact that, even at times of great challenge and distress, individuals noted how they had gained new self-understanding and reframed the way in which they perceived their life. Remaining open to such an 'attitude' when supporting others may therefore be of benefit.

Reflective questions

- How might an attitude of *'learning from experience'* fit with my understanding of crisis?
- Has anyone I have worked with reported spirituality as being either supportive or a barrier to their well-being and recovery?
- Did my response acknowledge or negate their experience and their perception of the situation?
- Was support available that enabled them to either enhance the effect (if it was supportive) or lessen the impact (if it was a barrier)?

Children's spirituality

People sometimes question whether children have a spiritual life but it is reasonable to assume that children are just as spiritual as adults. Clearly, as children are getting to know themselves and the world around them, the way they explore and experience spirituality needs to be considered in terms of their age, using developmentally appropriate methods. It would seem logical that the developmental milestones of childhood will include steps on the spiritual journey.

In support of the above statement, research suggests that children do experience and find ways to express their sense of spirituality; this is true of children from all cultures and spiritual/religious backgrounds, and it is 'largely spontaneous and natural' (Nye 2011, p.221). As with adults, it seems that spirituality helps children find meaning in their experiences. It can also offer them a method of coping with day-to-day challenges and gaining a sense of connection with themselves and those around them. They may be introduced to particular organised approaches to expressing spirituality, but they also draw on wider experiences as they explore their world (Walker 2005, Culliford 2011, Nye 2011, Clarke 2013).

If we are to work effectively with children, we need to integrate approaches that are suited to their developmental needs and personal preferences, which will enable them to explore and communicate their wishes in relation to spirituality. Aspects of spirituality may find their way into all manner of experiences, including death and other forms of loss, abuse, neglect, illness, family breakdown, cultural upheaval and war, as well as more constructive experiences that enliven a child's curiosity, compassion, and sense of awe in relation to the world around them. As with adult mental health, studies have noted a connection between reactions to all these experiences and spirituality, both in terms of risk and resilience (Peteet *et al.* 2011).

Unfortunately, there is a paucity of information regarding children and spirituality within health and social care professions, such as nursing; and what is available mostly focuses on 'religion' and 'dying' (Murphy *et al.* 2015). It is therefore important to develop a wider pool of resources to support all health and social care professionals working in this field. Forums such as the Spirituality and Psychiatry Special Interest Group (Royal College of Psychiatrists) and BACP Spirituality (British Association of Counselling and Psychotherapy) are excellent sources of information. Moreover, guidelines relating to professional groups such as occupational therapy, where spirituality (as an aspect of holistic practice) is considered to be a core value, can also prove useful (Hemphill 2015).

Reflective questions

- Reflecting on my childhood, can I recall experiences that I consider to be 'spiritual'? If so, what sensations, thoughts and 'sense of the moment' do I remember?
- From my current perspective, what do these childhood experiences mean? Do I consider these to be positive or negative experiences? Are they similar to experiences I have had as an adult or are they different? What have these experiences left me with?
- Did I share these experiences with others? If so, what was their response and how did this help or hinder my understanding? What else, if anything, may have been helpful at that time?

Spirituality and end of life care

One experience shared by all is that of death. Nearing this phase of existence, or spending time with others who are, may 'rekindle or intensify spiritual and religious concerns, or both' (Candy *et al.* 2009, p.1). This may include returning to previously introduced or explored beliefs which frame living and dying within particular spiritual teachings, or it may involve seeking out unexplored systems and narratives in an attempt to make sense of such experiences. Alternatively, or in addition, it may mean reflecting on issues such as relationships formed, actions taken, words spoken, losses mourned, opportunities missed, adventures completed, and many other aspects of life through which an individual perceives where they are in relation to their past, present and future. Preparing for the end of life can bring with it a wide range of feelings and responses, including uncertainty, fear, confusion, anger, and a conviction that there is more to do. Alternatively, it may bring relief, acceptance, and a readiness to let go. Although it is a collective existential experience, death is also highly personal in the way we each experience it and may wish to approach it.

When caring for individuals as they, or those they are close to, near the end of life, it is vitally important to create opportunities for them to reflect on, prepare for, and communicate their wishes relating to how they are feeling and what they would like to happen. This may include facilitating advance decision-making ('living will') processes regarding treatment as well as spiritual and other needs, all of which may or may not be intrinsically linked. Factors that individuals may wish to explore include their hopes, fears and expectations prior to, during and after death. Gauging the speed at which this might happen requires great sensitivity as well as courage on the practitioner's part, sensitivity regarding how and when to broach the subject, and stamina to 'stay with' whatever the experience brings for the individual and those around them.

Times such as these may also lead to difficult emotions and experiences being brought to the surface for the practitioner, which will require self-awareness, resilience and an openness to the concept of self-care, along with an understanding of how the practitioner's own beliefs around death, if not acknowledged and worked with, may intrude upon the experience of those they are caring for. All of this, along with treatment choices and palliative care support, inform quality of life experiences and go some way towards offering a 'whole person' response. Incorporating a level of spiritual competence within health and social care practitioner training will enhance the practitioner's ability to promote and deliver an optimal level of spiritual care during end of life.

Reflective questions

- When considering spirituality and end of life, what are my expectations, hopes and fears, and where might these ideas stem from?
- How comfortable do I feel about discussing end of life issues with individuals facing this experience? Are there any aspects I might find particularly difficult?
- If working with someone who chooses not to follow a potentially life-prolonging medical treatment due to it contravening their spiritual beliefs, how might I feel about this choice?

Perils, pitfalls and abuses of power: the harmful side of spirituality

Although research and practice suggest that a great deal of good can come from creating opportunities to explore and express spirituality, it can also bring distress and the potential for harm. On occasions, the underlying beliefs of a particular spiritual system can place pressure on individuals and groups to think and act in ways they find challenging or that result in difficult feelings, such as shame and low self-worth. Studies have also highlighted problems arising from being a member of destructive and dysfunctional groups (Gilbert & Parkes 2011). In addition, certain practices, although designed for purposes of personal and spiritual growth, may in themselves open people up to destabilisation or disorientation (Wright 2005). Such experiences may have a negative influence on well-being.

With regard to abuses of power, concerns have been raised as to how an individual or group might use spirituality to control, harm or meet their own distorted needs. Spiritual abuse has become high profile and all too common. It has ranged from one individual controlling another, through to leaders of small to medium-sized groups, to vast internationally based organisations where the abuse of members by clergy and other faith leaders has been ignored or, on occasions, deliberately hidden from view. Using spirituality for abusive means can impact greatly on the individual and wider group members, and those affected will therefore require sensitive, if not specialist, support.

Research and clinical work undertaken with survivors of cults and other abusive groups highlight the importance of understanding how deeply traumatising such experiences can be. We also need to understand how abusive individuals and groups utilise spirituality to control, groom and manipulate their victims (Orlowski 2010, Jenkinson 2013, Oakley & Kinmond 2013). The following is a broad definition of spiritual abuse proposed by Oakley and Kinmond (2013, p.21):

> SA [spiritual abuse] is coercion and control of one individual by another in a spiritual context. The target experiences SA as a deeply emotional personal attack ... [and] may include: manipulation and exploitation, enforced accountability, censorship of decision making, requirements for secrecy and silence, pressure to conform, misuse of scripture or the pulpit to control behaviour, requirement of obedience to the abuser, the suggestion that the abuser has a 'divine' position and isolation from others, especially those external to the abusive context.

These are important issues to consider when individuals are referred to health and social care services, whether they are victims or perpetrators. Referrals may relate to first generation members (those who have entered a cult or other such group at a later age) or second generation (those who have been born into or spent a majority of their life in such a group and therefore are likely to have limited experience of alternative ways of relating to others and the wider world). Spiritual abuse related policies and procedures have started to be developed (Oakley & Kinmond 2014), along with good practice guidelines to help professionals assess the support required by individuals and families who have experienced negative aspects of spirituality. There is growing awareness of how extensive such experiences have become, and it would therefore seem wise to invest further in this area of work.

Professional practice and workplace considerations

Personal awareness, practitioner care and workplace well-being

Health and social care are rewarding but complex and demanding areas of work and self-awareness and resilience are therefore vital. In addition, strategies need to be put in place that allow work to be undertaken in health-promoting ways over a long period of time. With this in mind, it is important to consider how practitioner beliefs and experiences inform and influence the work undertaken, as well as how the work impacts upon the practitioner.

Reflective questions

- What might happen, from both a personal and professional perspective, if opportunities to enhance my self-awareness and resilience are not created?
- How might spirituality underpin my self-care plans?

Health and social care professionals regularly come into close contact with individuals and families who have experienced trauma. Working in this field involves supporting these people as they find ways to cope with and move through the immediate and longer-term impact of a difficult/traumatic experience. Each practitioner's particular remit will define how this is done, but an essential ingredient in all such support is the 'relationship'.

With relationships come attachment styles and levels of empathic engagement. Although essential when working with others, the latter brings with it the potential of trauma being internalised by the practitioner – a phenomenon commonly known as *vicarious* or *secondary trauma*. Witnessing trauma through personal stories can impact on how professionals view themselves and others, along with their sense of safety, humanity and efficacy (Sanderson 2013). Signs and symptoms can manifest in similar ways to those experienced by the individuals supported, including high levels of stress and burnout. Such manifestations can ripple out into professional teams, organisations and practice settings. This includes situations where spirituality is in some way caught up with the trauma, or is not acknowledged in a health-promoting manner.

It is essential that appropriate support is in place for individual practitioners and wider teams. This ensures that the potential psychological disturbance and vicarious trauma caused by the work is held, reflected upon, and dissipated so the impact is short-lived and does not lead to individuals and teams becoming overwhelmed.

It is also important to remember the potential for spirituality to facilitate resilience and restoration, and this is relevant to health and social care professionals and service users alike. As spirituality is 'the solid centre in our lives that enables us to express ourselves in the world and to cope with all the complexities and conflicts of being alive' (Wright 2005, p.3), encouraging practitioners to draw from it, in whatever way suits their unique preferences and needs, can help to create a protective buffer. In addition, ensuring that adequate time and appropriate spaces are made available, a compassionate ethos is promoted, related programmes are unambiguously written into future workforce strategies, and the practitioner is respectfully acknowledged as a 'whole person'. All this would appear essential when promoting well-being in the workplace. In turn, practitioners will be better able to untangle themselves from the impact of the work they do, which consequently can help them do the *work better for longer*.

Spiritual competency

In their text, *Spiritual & Religious Competencies in Clinical Practice*, Vieten and Scammell (2015) outline competencies which they suggest are essential for psychologists and mental health professionals. However, it might be argued that such competencies are relevant to all who work within health and social care contexts. These competencies fall within three main domains, attitudes, knowledge and skills, and incorporate a range of elements, such as (adapted from Vieten & Scammell 2015, p.XV–XVI):

- empathy, respect, appreciation of diversity, awareness of how practitioner beliefs and backgrounds influence practice and processes
- understanding of different forms of spirituality; how spirituality and religion can both overlap and be distinct; taking a variety of experiences and difficulties into account when attempting to differentiate between psychopathological and other symptoms, along with lifespan changes, internal and external resources derived from spirituality, the potential for negative impact on health and well-being, and legal and ethical considerations
- the importance of acknowledging spirituality, strengths, resources and spiritual and religious problems when exploring a person's history, as well as remaining aware of current developments and research, recognising limitations regarding qualifications and competence, and the potential need to collaborate, consult and refer to appropriate others.

From a generic perspective, the above are not so different from other current professional guidelines, although, as noted elsewhere in this chapter, concerns remain with regard to holding a spiritual focus and applying this to practice. When it is included, it is often done in a somewhat peripheral manner, or assumptions are made as to what spirituality means (e.g. identifying it with religiosity), rather than allowing for broader possibilities.

Concerns have also been raised regarding pathologising certain spiritual beliefs and experiences. Although some practitioners claim to be open to including spirituality to some degree, they may be fearful that speaking of such things may have an 'anti-therapeutic effect' (Parkes & Barber 2011, p.124), or that, by allowing a space for spirituality, they are in some way crossing professional boundaries. The latter is intriguing when considering other potentially sensitive areas professionals are encouraged, if not expected, to explore as they gain a sense of the 'whole person' they are working with.

The importance of acknowledging spirituality, along with potential benefits and caveats, is evident. Such an acknowledgement also helps create a reflective space where things that provide meaning and purpose in a person's life can be explored. It would therefore seem fitting to review current practice, training programmes, professional guidelines, legislation and wider literature in order to offer truly holistic health and social care services.

Coming full circle: 'whole person' practice and concluding remarks

Spirituality is clearly a complex, multifaceted, challenging, yet important issue to consider in health and social care. A bio-psycho-social model is no longer sufficient; to gain a truly 'whole person' perspective, that which might be considered 'spiritual' needs to be added. As stated by Pilgrim (2014, p.72), spirituality 'offers a fourth dimension' to be added to a model that might be 'sufficient for materialists and atheists' but not enough for those who draw upon spirituality as a 'potential source of hope' and protection with regard to issues such as mental health.

Therefore, in addition to professionals exploring their own perspective and ways of expressing spirituality, the services in which they are based would be well advised to take into consideration this much-needed but greatly misunderstood and ignored dimension when designing, staffing and implementing services. If we fail to include the spiritual dimension, there is a risk of harming, rather than helping, those who both utilise and work within health and social care. As noted by Jenkins (2011, p.29):

> … because spirituality is at the heart of how people understand themselves in the world, an attack on someone's spirituality or its denial is an attack on the heart of the person, on their integrity, their wholeness. To refuse to take someone's spirituality seriously is to refuse to take them seriously. To seek to convince someone that precisely what helps them hold themselves together is 'immature', 'psychotic', in need of medicating away or has no place in their healing is to do great violence.

In this chapter, we have explored many facets of spirituality in relation to health and social care, ranging from what it is, to how important it might be, its relevance in a variety of contexts, how it might be harmful, its applicability to practitioner care and workplace well-being, and its place in 'whole person' practice. Whether we are experienced practitioners who have chosen to use this book to support and train others, or trainees or newly qualified professionals launching ourselves into our new role, it seems appropriate to assess how well we, and the services we work within, acknowledge and facilitate a space for spirituality. The challenge is ours.

Reflective questions

- In what ways and how well is spirituality acknowledged within the organisation in which I currently work or hope to work in the future?
- How does this help or hinder my own and the service's capacity to support others?
- In relation to spirituality, what would I like to see done differently, if anything, to enhance the service offered and to support me in my work?

References

BACP Spirituality. http://bacpspirituality.org.uk/ (last accessed 27.12.2016).

BPS Division of Counselling Psychology Spirituality Special Interest Group: http://www.bps.org.uk/networks-and-communities/member-microsite/division-counselling-psychology/spirituality (last accessed 27.12.2016).

Brett, C.M.C. (2010). 'Transformative crises' in I. Clarke (ed.) *Psychosis and Spirituality: Consolidating the New Paradigm.* 2nd edn. Chichester: Wiley.

Candy, B., Jones, L., Speck, P., Tookman, A. & King, M. (2009). *Spiritual and Religious Interventions for Adults in the Terminal Phase of Disease.* Chichester: John Wiley & Sons Ltd.

Clarke, I. (2010). *Psychosis and Spirituality: Consolidating a New Paradigm.* 2nd edn. Chichester: John Wiley & Sons Ltd.

Clarke, J. (2013). *Spiritual Care in Everyday Nursing Practice: A New Approach.* Hampshire: Palgrave Macmillan.

Culliford, L. (2011). *The Psychology of Spirituality: An Introduction.* London: Jessica Kingsley Publishers.

Department of Health (DH) (2011). *No Health Without Mental Health: A Cross-Government Mental Health Outcomes Strategy for People of All Ages.* London: DH.

Gilbert, P. (2011). *Spirituality and Mental Health.* Brighton: Pavilion Publishing Ltd.

Gilbert, P. & Parkes, M. (2011). *Report on the place of spirituality in mental health.* London: The National Spirituality and Mental Health Forum.

Hemphill, B. (2015). Spiritual assessments in Occupational Therapy. *The Open Journal of Occupational Therapy.* **3** (3), 1–16.

Holloway, M. & Moss, B. (2010). *Spirituality and Social Work.* London: Palgrave Macmillan.

Jenkins, C. (2011). 'When client's spirituality is denied in therapy' in W. West (ed.) *Exploring Therapy, Spirituality and Healing.* Hampshire: Palgrave MacMillan. 28–47.

Jenkinson, G. (2013). Working with cult survivors. *Therapy Today.* **24** (4), 18–21.

Kaminker, J. & Lukoff, D. (2013) 'Transpersonal perspectives on mental health' in H.L. Friedman & G. Hartelius (eds) *The Wiley Blackwell Handbook of Transpersonal Psychology.* Sussex: John Wiley and Sons Ltd. 417–32.

King, M., Marston, L., McManus, S., Brugha, T., Meltzer, H. & Bebbington, P. (2013). Religion, spirituality and mental health: results from a national study of English households. *British Journal of Psychiatry.* **202**, 68–73.

Koenig, H.G. (2013). *Spirituality in Patient Care: Why, How, When, and What.* Pennsylvania: Templeton Press.

Koenig, H.G., King, D.E. & Benner Carson, V. (2012). *Handbook for Religion and Health.* 2nd edn. Oxford: Oxford University Press.

Lukoff, D., Turner, R. & Lu, F.G. (1993). Transpersonal psychology research review: Psychospiritual dimensions and healing. *Journal of Transpersonal Psychology.* **25**, (1), 11–28.

Lukoff, D., Lu, F.G. & Yang, M.D. (2011). 'DSM-1V Religious and spiritual problems' in J.R. Peteet *et al.* (eds) *Religious and Spiritual Issues in Psychiatric Diagnosis: A Research Agenda for DSM-V.* Virginia: American Psychiatric Publishing Inc.

McSherry, W. & Ross, L. (2015). A spiritual shortfall? *Nursing Standard.* **29**, (35), 22.

Moore, T. (1998). *Care of the Soul: How to Add Depth and Meaning to your Everyday Life.* New York: HarperCollins Publishers Inc.

Murphy, M.M., Begley, T., Timmins, F., Neill, F. & Sheaf, G. (2015). Spirituality and spiritual care – missing concepts from core undergraduate children's nursing textbooks. *International Journal of Children's Spirituality.* **20** (2), 114–28.

Nye, R. (2011). 'Children's and young people's well-being' in P. Gilbert (ed.) *Spirituality and Mental Health.* Brighton: Pavilion Publishing Ltd.

Oakley, L. & Kinmond, K. (2013). *Breaking the Silence on Spiritual Abuse.* Hampshire: Palgrave Macmillan.

Oakley, L.R. & Kinmond, K.S. (2014). Developing safeguarding policy and practice for spiritual abuse. *The Journal of Adult Protection.* **16** (2), 87–95.

O'Connell, K.A. & Skevington, S.M. (2010). Spiritual, religious, and personal beliefs are important and distinctive to assessing quality of life in health: A comparison of theoretical models. *British Journal of Health Psychology.* **15**, 729–48.

Orlowski, B.M. (2010). *Spiritual Abuse Recovery: Dynamic research on finding a place of wholeness.* Oregon: Wipf & Stock.

Parkes, M. & Barber, J. (2011). 'Professional attitudes' in P. Gilbert (ed.) *Spirituality and Mental Health.* Brighton: Pavilion Publishing Ltd.

Peteet, J.R., Lu, F.G. & Narrow, W.E. (2011). *Religious and Spiritual Issues in Psychiatric Diagnosis: A Research Agenda for DSM-V.* Virginia: American Psychiatric Publishing Inc.

Pilgrim, D. (2014). *Key Concepts in Mental Health.* 3rd edn. London: SAGE.

Rohricht, F., Basdekis-Jozsa, R., Sidhu, J., Mukhtar, A., Suzuki, L. & Priebe, S. (2009). The association of religiosity spirituality, and ethnic background with ego-pathology in acute schizophrenia. *Mental Health, Religion & Culture.* **12** (6), 515–26.

Royal College of Psychiatrists (2011). *Recommendations for psychiatrists on spirituality and religion: position statement.* London: Royal College of Psychiatrists.

Royal College of Psychiatrists Spirituality and Psychiatry Special Interest Group. http://www.rcpsych.ac.uk/workinpsychiatry/specialinterestgroups/spirituality.aspx (last accessed 27.12.2016).

Sanderson, C. (2013). *Counselling Skills for Working with Trauma: Healing from Child Sexual Abuse, Sexual Violence and Domestic Abuse.* London: Jessica Kingsley Publishers.

Spiritual Competency Resource Center. http://www.spiritualcompetency.com/ (last accessed 27.12.2016).

Spiritual Crisis Network website. http://spiritualcrisisnetwork.uk/ (last accessed 27.12.2016).

Swinton, J. (2001). *Spirituality and Mental Health Care: Rediscovering the 'Forgotten' Dimension.* London: Jessica Kingsley Publishers.

Vieten, C. & Scammell, S. (2015). *Spiritual & Religious Competencies in Clinical Practice: Guidelines for Psychotherapists & Mental Health Professionals*. California: New Harbinger Publications Inc.

Walker, S. (2005). *Culturally Competent Therapy: Working with Children and Young People.* Hampshire: Palgrave Macmillan.

Welsh Government (2010). *Standards for Spiritual Care Services in the NHS in Wales 2010*. Cardiff: Welsh Government.

West, W. (2011). *Exploring Therapy, Spirituality and Healing.* Hampshire: Palgrave Macmillan.

Wright, S.G. (2005). *Reflections on Spirituality and Health*. London: Whurr Publishers Ltd.

Chapter 15

The resilient practitioner: working in a context of change

Stuart Abbott

Learning outcomes
By the end of this chapter you will be able to:
- Understand the importance of resilience and how it impacts on health and well-being
- Link resilience in practice to caring for clients/patients safely and compassionately
- Have the knowledge and understanding to develop personal resilience in order to enhance your own practice and well-being
- Recognise the link between resilience and professional competency and duty of care.

Introduction
Given the inherent emotional demands of their jobs and the almost constant changes faced by health and social care professionals, resilience (as both a theoretical concept and practical attribute) is of key significance. This applies not only to practitioners who are about to enter the sector or at an early career stage, but also to those who have had to deal with constant change, heavy workloads and pressure to meet increasingly challenging performance-driven targets.

Practitioner resilience is not an innate trait or talent but rather an aspect of ongoing personal and professional development, comprising a range of skills, attributes, attitudes and behaviours that can be learnt and developed. This chapter will therefore provide the reader with an overview of resilience and also highlight applied approaches that individuals can utilise in order to develop resilience within their own professional context.

Defining practitioner resilience

Resilience can broadly be defined as a capacity to overcome and recover positively from adversity. It is appropriate to note the complexities involved in defining the concept. Grant and Kinman suggest the term 'resilience' should be understood as an umbrella term which constitutes a 'diverse range of competencies, capacities and behaviours that not only help people to manage adversity, but gain strength from such experiences' (2014a, p.19). Research into the concept from across a diverse range of social science disciplines highlights the complex and contextual nature of resilience (Southwick *et al.* 2014). There are many different models of resilience but they all view it as the outcome of a process, acknowledging its changeable, dynamic and context- specific nature.

In offering her synthesis of a range of literature examining the construct, Waller defines it as 'a multidetermined and ever-changing product of interacting forces within a given ecosystemic context' (2001, p.290). Central to this definition is the idea of resilience as a dynamic outcome of a variable system of interrelated influences; a quality that contemporary specialists in the field have agreed on in recent years (e.g. Luthar *et al.* 2000, Southwick *et al.* 2014, Grant & Kinman 2014b, Masten 2014).

The word 'ecosystemic' denotes the holistic nature of the interplay between individual and environmental factors in influencing the outcome of emotional resilience. The dynamic and systemic contexts for resilience are relevant to the present discussion in that they draw attention to a dichotomy of influence upon practitioner resilience. Firstly, there is the changing and developing experience of the individual practitioner – resilience is, in itself, a product of the changing and temporal nature of human emotional experience. Secondly, there is the range of external conditions that influence human emotional experience. The most important of these for our discussion is the personal context of the practitioner, the nature of practice and patient interrelation, and the organisational or workplace environment in which the practitioner operates. This complex interrelationship of factors determines and influences the extent to which a practitioner feels able, and has the emotional and practical capacity, to overcome occupational adversity in its varying forms, and respond proactively in order to continue their personal and professional development.

In order to understand the concept of resilience, we need to recognise the practitioner's affective domain, of which resilience can be said to be one aspect: it is in fact a human emotional response to adversity. By locating the notion of resilience within the sphere of individual human emotional experience, a practitioner can approach the development of emotional resilience as something that can be understood, cultivated and applied as a personal and occupational attribute and perhaps, to an extent, 'mastered' as a professional competency. As a multifaceted and changeable attribute that can be learnt through an understanding of the self and the individual's experience within their occupational context, resilience can be cultivated and realised through a range of skills, behaviours, strategies and approaches that centre upon the development of emotional self-awareness in personal and professional contexts.

As you would expect, various characteristics of resilient people and qualities of resilience have been identified within academic literature. For our purposes, these can be grouped as follows. Firstly, such individuals have a strong self-awareness comprising a sense of emotional intelligence, self-efficacy, self-esteem, autonomy, identity, social confidence, self-compassion and empathy. Secondly, they follow a set of strategic behaviours such as future orientation, problem identification and solving. Finally, creativity, decision making, resourcefulness and a coherent outlook all provide these individuals with the means to be flexible and adaptable in their approach to overcoming change and challenge within professional practice.

Reflective questions

- What do you understand by the terms 'multidetermined' and 'ecosystemic' in relation to the concept of resilience?
- Consider your personal qualities of resilience in terms of your own levels of self-awareness, strategic behaviours, creativity, decision making, resourcefulness and coherence.
- What have you learned about your strengths and needs in terms of your personal qualities and resilience?

Challenges to resilience within the health and social care sector

Nature of helping professions

Helping professions are, by their nature, emotionally demanding. Being care based, they require the practitioner to give something of their 'self' to others; this may be in emotional or practical terms, or most often both (see Chapter 13 for more on this). A broad body of research conducted on health care professionals has found high rates of 'burnout', work-related stress, vicarious trauma and compassion fatigue amongst helping professionals (Beddoe *et al.* 2013, Clouston 2015, Grant & Kinman 2014b) (see Chapters 13 and 14 for more on this). Furthermore, a range of individual and organisational work-related stressors have been identified. These include having to manage uncertain, complex situations; lack of control, emotionally demanding interaction with patients;

lack of supporting structures; working within publicly scrutinised environments; and burgeoning caseloads, to name a few (Skovholdt & Trotter-Mathison 2011, Adamson *et al.* 2012; Grant & Kinman 2014b).

A second challenge to the practitioner (and this is particularly true of service providers within the NHS) is almost continual organisational change, mainly manifested through the implementation of new managerial and target-driven structures and systems. These changes often seek to streamline, quantify and risk-manage practice, and can result in conflicting demands being placed upon the practitioner and their engagement with patients/clients. This culminates in a distancing of the relationship between practitioner and patient, which, in turn inhibits the practitioner's ability to act according to their own intuitive values; instead they are forced to behave in accordance with the systemic demands imposed upon them (Scholes 2008).

Early career stages

A major challenge for those in the early stages of a career in health and social care is lack of experience in addressing emotional and organisational adversity within a workplace environment. Initial experiences of such difficulty can be particularly testing, as early career professionals lack the tacit and intuitive knowledge gained from having previously overcome adversity, and are also deficient in the confidence gained from the internalised realisation that they are, indeed, capable (Skovholdt & Rønnestad 2003).

Balance throughout the career

The notion of 'balance' between the various domains or contexts of one's experience is vital to the well-being of an individual, and a sense of balance helps one proactively address adversity. However, striking such a balance is often easier said than done, given the intense competing demands individuals endure in the various roles they occupy in modern personal and professional life. These roles and demands are of course ever changing in their nature for health and social care workers at any point of their career – and those embarking on professional experience in particular.

It is important to focus on balance as a contributory factor to personal well-being and an influential aspect of the development of resilience: an individual is better placed to address and overcome adversity when feeling more prepared in themselves, in the situation in which they find themselves. An imbalance between personal and professional life can result in increased or disproportionate demands being made of an individual in a given domain. This results in a drain on resilience across all domains or the individual experiencing decreased capacity to address the demands of the whole (Clouston 2014, 2015). Such issues may manifest as depression, anxiety and physical health problems, coupled with a sense of greater adversity within one's professional practice.

Competencies informing practitioner resilience
Adaptability and flexibility

The main quality needed to address and positively overcome adversity is the ability to adapt appropriately in situations that require a resilient response. This may simply mean being able to consider an apparent problem or issue from a different angle that better enables one to avoid or mitigate potential negative impacts. Alternatively, it could require a more complex and fundamental re-evaluation of personal values, attitudes and beliefs in order to overcome complex adversity that emotionally challenges an individual's conception of themselves.

The capacity to recognise the need for change, and to implement the change required, is also fundamental in developing practitioner resilience. As an aspect of self-awareness, flexibility enables the practitioner to better read and understand both their own emotional reactions and those of their patients /clients. This is key, since it enables meaningful positive relationships to be built that provide sustainable support for all concerned. The ability to 'flex', 'bend' or adapt is not merely practical; it also applies to the very heart of emotional experience in professional practice. If we become too 'rigid' or forthright in affective matters in professional practice, we risk adding further stress to already taut and challenging situations; it is therefore in a practitioner's interest to be prepared to adapt and bend in order to accommodate and/or 'brush off' emotionally draining experiences, as appropriate to the individual's well-being.

The ability to adapt and be flexible is also intimately bound up with attributes such as self-efficacy and autonomy; the ability to decide to be flexible in the face of change in adverse situations contributes towards an increased sense of emotional security, reliance, confidence and, ultimately, a greater resilience when encountering practice-based challenges.

Reflective questions

- Can you identify a time when you used an adaptable and flexible approach in a challenging situation? If not, can you think of situation where you *could* have used such an approach?
- What was the outcome of that situation? Or, if you imagine that you applied these principles, what would have been the outcome of that situation?
- What are your thoughts and feelings about adopting a flexible and adaptable approach in difficult situations?

Emotional intelligence

Emotional life (just like maths or reading) can be handled with greater or lesser skill, and requires a unique set of competencies. And how adept a person is at those is crucial to understanding why one person thrives in life while another, of equal intellect, dead-ends: emotional aptitude is a *meta-ability* (Goleman 1996, p.36).

Emotional awareness (which contributes towards emotional resilience) is recognised as being central to the attributes required by a successful practitioner within the helping professions. Research has shown that individuals displaying increased emotional intelligence are more adaptable, flexible, confident, better able to solve problems, make decisions, co-operate in collaborative environments, identify and implement appropriate coping mechanisms, develop professionally and enhance their own individual well-being (George 2000, Howe 2008).

Empathy

Empathy is fundamental to the practitioner in patient/client relationships on several levels. Primarily, the practitioner must have the capacity to consider the impact the adversity experienced by the patient or client has had on them, as individuals. As a core attribute for those in helping professions, empathy also poses a risk to the practitioner; excessive empathy can place too great an emotional burden on the practitioner, resulting in 'compassion fatigue' or 'emotional burnout' (Clouston 2015). Empathic relationships should therefore be observed, reflected upon and learnt from – so that they remain balanced and healthy for the practitioner. This will prevent such emotional activity detracting from their personal well-being. Through the development of a reflective self-awareness, empathy and the benefits and costs that it brings can be better understood, thus enabling practitioners to engage with patients/clients emotionally whilst also safeguarding themselves against negative impacts.

Approaches to the development of practitioner resilience

Self-awareness

Key to constructing professional resilience is an awareness of self, an ongoing understanding of one's own emotional, spiritual and practical make-up. Cultivating self-awareness requires practitioners to become more aware of their own value systems, motivations, aversions and aspirations – in order to develop a greater understanding of the personal self, and thus become more perceptive regarding what they are capable and incapable of, and what they will, and will not, accept (Jack & Smith 2007). Such introspection can be challenging at first: contemporary social and educational systems traditionally give us little opportunity to become accustomed to such approaches; and this is then accentuated by the fact that our busy lives often leave little time for effective contemplation of self (Clouston 2015).

It is therefore important that practitioners make an effort to develop self-awareness and associated emotional intelligence in order to become more resilient in the workplace. An understanding of self is intimately bound up with emotional intelligence: to be self-aware is to recognise one's own affective strengths and limitations. For those in the helping professions, it is vital to acknowledge the extent to which they are able to empathise with others (namely the patient/client in a professional context) before excessive empathy has a detrimental impact on them. Development of self-awareness, like resilience, is an ongoing and dynamic process: it changes as we change. This may be in response to positive or negative life experiences (either in a practitioner's personal life or as a reaction to the buffeting and stress of challenge and change in the professional environment). Engaging in an increased awareness of self is a key facet of the active and conscious development of practitioner resilience; thus the following approaches all contribute to this process.

Reflective practice

Constructive reflection upon one's professional practice provides a foundation for personal and professional development of resilience within the workplace. Through consideration of personal values, strengths, weaknesses, decisions, reactions and impacts, a practitioner is better able to identify and cultivate appropriate competencies relevant to their personal well-being and professional practice. In addressing the positive and adverse experiences that practice presents, from a critical, impartial and observational perspective, a more self-protective and practice-aware approach can be engendered. Constructive reflection is an effective means of developing self-awareness, emotional intelligence and empathy. Through critical insight, practitioners are better able to examine their own emotional dynamic within personal, practice and workplace contexts.

Grant and Kinman (2014c) highlight the benefits of group narrative reflection, presenting a technique to be used by practitioners engaged in patient/client relationships and citing its potential for increased empathic reflection and reflective communication. With a developed personal understanding gained from reflection, the practitioner can relate professional experience and practice to theory and vice versa. This process is vital in order to gain an increased understanding of what becoming a resilient professional practitioner entails.

Having placed the lived experience of practice within the reflective learning cycle of critical observation, analysis and theorising and then enacting a resulting positive intervention within practice, a practitioner is better positioned to observe and learn from experience and refine their professional practice accordingly. Through increased awareness of their own personal and professional experience, they can develop greater confidence, efficacy and autonomy in decision-making as a health and social care professional.

Supervision and coaching

Applying the reflective process within a professional learning setting benefits the practitioner in many ways. Key among these is the opportunity to consider professional practice and its emotional impact with others who have had similar experiences and can offer advice. However, the supervisory process is also a crucial means of developing an individual's practitioner identity and its associated respect or regard within professional social contexts. Supervision and coaching prompt and enable the reflective process in contextually rich and meaningful ways with learning occurring at the personal, practice and organisational levels. They provide opportunities to explore the experience of practice and receive occupational support in a safe and confidence-building environment.

Central to such professional support is the consideration and sharing of experience as a proven strategy for overcoming the challenges of the emotional and affective experiences faced in practice. Such tools and approaches are vital in building understanding of, and resilience to, the emotionally transactional, empathic relationship between practitioner and patient/client. Those working in the helping professions should therefore routinely engage in reflective supervision, as the application of the reflective cycle as an organisational tool results in the positive adaptation of practice – to the benefit of practitioners, patients/clients and the workplace as a whole.

Internal locus of control

Internal locus of control is essentially the recognition that an individual is in control of their own purpose and the subsequent use of this understanding to be proactive in one's behaviour for the benefit of self and/or others. The belief that one is responsible for one's own accomplishments is, in itself, a key driver towards ongoing personal and professional development. In addition, it provides a level of confidence within, and thus resilience towards, adverse or challenging situations.

Positive attributes that contribute to the development of an internal locus of control include: a sense of self-efficacy manifested through proactive decision-making, opportunity recognition, and an ability to negotiate and influence. As noted previously, a keen self-awareness regarding what is, and is not, controllable is central to developing effective behaviours. This may take the form of personal and emotional development as well as gaining the practical ability to implement small-scale change within the professional context that reduces workplace stressors and ideally gives more opportunity for resilience development.

Mindfulness

Mindfulness can be defined as the conscious effort to focus on the present moment without making judgements about related feelings or behaviours on the part of the practitioner or others. It is a means of observing, with little or no attachment to the situation in hand, thus allowing an insight into the present that is less tainted by emotion (Hanh 2010). Such observation can help the development of resilience as well as benefiting professional practice through enhanced emotional awareness, acceptance, objectivity, clarity, adaptability, concentration, self-control, self-compassion, empathy, communication and interpersonal skills and the ability to manage stress as well as increased psychological and physical health.

At its most fundamental, mindfulness enables a practitioner to be conscious of their reactions to whatever they are experiencing in the moment (Hanh 2010). Such reflection *within the moment* can contribute to a greater understanding of self, with the intention that our emotional responses will no longer drive us. Instead, we are able to observe our own responses and then make a conscious choice *not* to be governed by them. This can increase resilience by allowing a practitioner to recognise and avoid, or at least mitigate, potential emotional flashpoints that may occur within their practice.

Reflective questions

- Are you aware of any 'emotional flashpoints' in your everyday practice?
- Having read this chapter, how can you address or mitigate those flashpoints?
- Consider applying the strategies described in this chapter to enhance your self-awareness and support your resilience to help you with this.

Conclusion

This chapter has offered a definition of resilience as a theoretical concept and professional attribute, as applied within health and social care practice. Whilst recognising that the notion and indeed the attributes of practitioner resilience are multifaceted, complex, subjective and dependent on the context in which they are experienced, there are, nevertheless, various types of knowledge, behaviour and approach that can be considered as contributing to the development of an increased personal and professional resilience. These skills should be cultivated and employed with a view to developing practitioner resilience as an attribute of an evolving personal and professional practitioner identity. This can be achieved by engaging in what might be termed a process of personal and professional development involving constructive reflection on the self as it navigates the various roles and domains in which it engages. Through ongoing observation and iterative development of the emotional and personal self, a practitioner is better able to identify and address the needs and challenges faced by the professional self within a health and social care organisational workplace.

References

Adamson, C., Beddoe, L. & Davys, A. (2012). Building resilient practitioners: Definitions and practitioner understandings. *British Journal of Social Work*. **32** (1), 100–117.

Beddoe, L., Davys, A., and Adamson, C. (2013). Educating resilient practitioners. *Social Work Education*. **32** (1), 100–117.

Clouston, T.J. (2014). Whose occupational balance is it anyway? The challenge of neoliberal capitalism and work-life imbalance. *British Journal of Occupational Therapy*. **77** (10), 507–15.

Clouston, T.J. (2015). *Challenging Stress, Burnout and Rust-Out: Finding Balance in Busy Lives*. London: Jessica Kingsley.

George, J. (2000). Emotions and leadership: the role of emotional intelligence. *Human Relations*. **53**, 1027–55.

Goleman, D. (1996). *Emotional Intelligence*. London: Bloomsbury.

Grant, L. & Kinman, G. (2012). Enhancing well-being in social work students: Building resilience in the next generation. *Social Work Education*. **31**(5), 605–21.

Grant, L. & Kinman, G. (2014a). 'What is resilience?' in L. Grant & G. Kinman (eds) *Developing Resilience for Social Work Practice*. London: Palgrave Macmillan.

Grant, L. & Kinman, G. (2014b). *Developing Resilience for Social Work Practice*. London: Palgrave Macmillan.

Grant, L. & Kinman, G. (2014c). Emotional resilience in the helping professions and how it can be enhanced. *Health and Social Care Education*. **3** (1), 23–34.

Hanh, T.N. (2010). *You are Here: Discovering the Magic of the Present*. Boston, MA: Shambhala Publications.

Howe, D. (2008). *The Emotionally Intelligent Social Worker*. London: Palgrave Macmillan.

Jack, K. & Smith, A. (2007). Promoting self-awareness in nurses to improve nursing practice. *Nursing Standard*. **21** (32), 47–52.

Luthar, S.S., Cicchetti, D. & Becker, B. (2000). The construct of resilience: A critical evaluation and guidelines for future work. *Child Development*. **71** (3), 543–62.

Masten, A.S. (2014). Global perspectives on resilience in children and youth. *Child Development*. **85** (1), 6–20.

Scholes, J. (2008). Why health care needs resilient practitioners. *Nursing in Critical Care*. **13** (6), 281–85.

Skovholt, T.M. & Rønnestad, M.H. (2003). Struggles of the novice counsellor and therapist. *Journal of Career Development*. **30** (1), 45–58.

Skovholt, T.M. & Trotter-Mathison, M. (2011). *The Resilient Practitioner: Burnout Prevention and Self-care Strategies for Counsellors, Therapists, Teachers and Health Professionals*. London: Routledge.

Southwick, S.M., Bonanno, G.A., Masten, A.S., Panter-Brick, C. & Yehuda, R. (2014). Resilience definitions, theory, and challenges: Interdisciplinary perspectives. *European Journal of Psychotraumatology*. **5**, 25338 http://dx.doi.org/10.3402/ejpt.v5.25338 (last accessed 22.9.2017).

Waller, M.A. (2001). Resilience in ecosystemic context: Evolution of the concept. *American Journal of Orthopsychiatry*. **71** (3), 290–97.

Epilogue:
Conclusions for the reader and the way forward

Steven W. Whitcombe, Lyn Westcott and Teena J. Clouston

This book has explored and reflected upon the skills and qualities necessary to meet the challenges and transitions we have to pass through in order to develop our 'professional selves' in practice. These multiple selves emerge over time; they build upon and learn from one another, and reflexively interact with the changing context, unique circumstances and factors that influence each individual at any point in time.

Having read the book, you will understand that these different strands cannot be looked at in isolation, because they are so interconnected; instead they all contribute to a complex and dynamic system of integrated health and social care, which is in a constant state of change and evolution. Throughout the chapters, the authors have highlighted how transitions at all levels of practice, are affected by personal, professional, organisational and political agendas that create critical challenges. They have also identified how you can interact with and confront these to effect positive action and change.

There are two crucial lessons we hope you will take forward as a result of engaging with this text. Firstly, you need to develop the ability to recognise how these external and, indeed, internal forces influence your personal and professional journey in terms of coping well with transitions. Secondly, you need to consider and understand how the techniques and theories herein can help you to develop and/or adapt your ability to cope with these everyday challenges and critical incidents. This, we hope, will enhance your ability to achieve and sustain successful transitions in practice and achieve the best outcome, not only for your patients/clients, but also for your own well-being and that of your colleagues.

Whilst no one can know the shape of health and social care services in the future, or the political drivers that will influence these, we can be aware of the skills we need to manage our interface with these transitions and thus ensure a smooth, professional and successful passage through them. This includes upholding key values like care, compassion and person-centred working, no matter what pressures are put upon you – although we do ask you to raise concerns about this! We hope this book has given you the knowledge and understanding to carefully consider the challenges and demands that you will meet, and respond to them in a way that upholds your professional values and personal integrity.

Whatever point you have reached on your journey, we wish you well with your career, and hope this book will play some part (however small) in your future achievements.

Index

6 Cs 184

abuse, emotional 157
abuse of vulnerable adults 140
abuse, physical 157
abuse, sexual 157
abuse, spiritual 198
accountability 20, 21
Act of Parliament 102
adult protection, history of 140
advanced beginners 37
advocacy 166
affective learning 34
Andrews Report 170
'any qualified provider' (AQP) 115
austerity 113, 122
autonomy 4, 45–54

Baby P 169
beneficence 4
breaking bad news 91, 92
burnout 52, 174, 207

Care and Social Services Inspectorate Wales CSSIW 105
care, culture of 171, 179
Care Inspectorate 106
care, models of 182, 183
Care Quality Commission (CQC) 104, 143, 146
caring values 165–185
caring values, definition of 166
change, coping with 53
child abuse 157–159
child in need, definition of 157
child labour 154
child protection
    (see also safeguarding children) 154, 155, 157
Children Act (1989) 155, 157
Children Act (2004) 156
child sexual exploitation (CSE) 158
clinical commissioning groups (CCGs) 115
clinical educator 118, 120
Clothier Inquiry 169
coaching 212
codes of conduct 5, 19, 147

commissioning service providers 116
committee stage 102
communication 22, 23, 62, 85–94
communication, changing context of 89
communication, forms of 85, 86
communication, professional expectations regarding 93
communication with carers 88
communication with colleagues 88
communication with patients 87
Community Care and Health (Scotland) Act (2002) 74
compassion 167
compassion fatigue 207
competence 38, 39
complaints 9
confidentiality 36, 88
conflict resolution 66
continuing professional development (CPD) 46, 48, 49, 50, 110
cost-effectiveness 114, 115
cost of running the NHS 114
courage 167

death and spirituality 196, 197
devolved powers 100
dignity 23, 37, 167
dress code 23
duty of candour ix, 10, 116, 144
duty to care 147

efficiency 119, 120
emotional engagement 38
emotional intelligence 210
empathy 167, 210
end-of-life care 196
England 73, 104
entrepreneurship 121, 122
ethical code 5, 147, 148
ethics 4
expertise 41, 42

failings in care 169, 170, 171
female genital mutilation (FGM) 158, 159, 161
fitness to practise (FTP) 9
Five Year Forward View 103

Francis Report ix, 116, 141, 143, 170
Freedom to Speak Up Guardians xiii, 12

Generation Y 19
governance 78
green papers 101

Haringey Serious Case Review 169
Health Act (1999) 73
Health and Care Professions Council (HCPC) 147
Health and Safety Executive (HSE) 104
Health and Social Care Bill (2012) 73
Health and Social Care Act (2013) 100, 102
Health and Social Care (Reform) Act (Northern Ireland) (2009) 74
health care assistants 121
Healthcare Improvement Scotland (HIS) 106
Healthcare Inspectorate Wales (HIW) 105

independent practice 38
inspectorates 107
integrity 167
internal markets 115
Internet use 90, 91
interpersonal conflict 65
interpretivist research paradigm 129, 130
interprofessional education 108
interprofessional working 117

John Lewis 17
journal club 132
justice 5

Laming Report 107, 156, 169
learning domains 34
learning journey 31–42
legal aspects of health care 99–111
legislative process 101, 102
locus of control, internal 212

market forces and health care 180

marketplace, health and social care as 114
Mental Capacity Act (2005) 145
mentoring 50, 51
mentorship, modern 51
Mid Staffordshire Hospital ix, x, 1, 100, 141
mindfulness 212, 213
Monitor (NHS) 105
moral compass 177, 178
multidisciplinary team 61, 62

National Health Services (Wales) Act (2006) 74
neglect 158
negligence 6
neoliberalism 180
NHS Act (2006) 73
NHS Constitution, principles and values 171, 172, 173
NHS Reform (Scotland) Act 2004 74
non-judgemental approach 168
non-maleficence 4
Northern Ireland 74, 105
novice to expert 32, 33
novices 35

online communication 93
organisational change and resilience 208

partnership working 71–82, 172
partnership working, barriers to 76, 77
partnership working, benefits of 75
partnership working legislation 73
partnership working, power relations in 77, 80
partnership working and service users and carers 81
patient-centred approach 116
personal appearance 23
person-centred approach 168, 179
policy documents 103
policy-making process 73
political aspects of health care 99–111
positive professional behaviour, impact of 21
positivism 129

postgraduate study 133
power 78, 80
practice, modes of 184
practitioner care 199
preceptorship 67
pre-registration programmes 47
professional associations 110
professional behaviour 17–28
professional competence model 183
professional curiosity 162
professional doctorate 134
professional ethics 3, 4, 177
professionals' interests 79
professional proficiency 8
professional qualification 46
professional registration 7, 8, 38, 110
professional standards and regulation 7, 47
Professional Standards Authority (PSA) 6
proficiency 39, 41
psychological contract 180
Public Bodies (Joint Working) (Scotland) Act 2014 74

raising concerns 11, 12, 149
Regulation and Quality Improvement Authority (RQIA) 105
regulatory bodies 6, 100, 104, 107, 109, 110, 143
reflective practice 211
research 127–135
research collaboration in the workplace 132
research, definition of 128
research paradigms 129, 130, 131
research skills, use of in practice 132
resilience 52, 53, 205–213
resilience and flexibility 209
resilience, challenges to in health and social care 207
resilience, definition of 206
resilient individuals, characteristics of 207
resources, reduction in 113
respect 24, 37, 168
respectful uncertainty 162
responsibility 20, 21
rule of optimism 162

safeguarding adults, principles of 146
safeguarding adults, statutory guidance on 144, 145
safeguarding children (see also child protection) 153–163
safeguarding children, organisational responsibilities in 160, 161
safeguarding training 160, 161
safeguarding vulnerable adults 139–150
science 128
Scotland 74, 106
self-awareness 210, 211
self-reflection on professional behaviour 26
Shipman, Harold 141, 169
skill acquisition 32, 33
Social Care and Social Work Improvement Scotland (SCSWIS) 106
social integration in teams 61
social media 36, 89, 90, 91
social media and professionalism 92
Social Services and Well-being Act (2014) 74
soul 191
SPIKES protocol 92
spiritual competency 200
spiritual crisis 194
spirituality 189–202
spirituality and end-of-life care 196, 197
spirituality and mental health 193, 194
spirituality, children's 195
spirituality, definitions of 189
spirituality, negative aspects of 197, 198
standards of conduct 7, 8
stress 52
students 10, 17
supervision 212

team development 64
team roles 63
team working 59–68, 88
trauma, vicarious 199, 207
trust 168

United Nations Convention on the
    Rights of the Child (UNCRC) 155
universities, research links with 133
unprofessional behaviour 20

value for money 173
values based recruitment 32, 177
values, personal 174, 176, 177
values, shared 180
vanguard sites 103
vulnerable adult, definition of 142, 143

Wales 74, 105
whistleblowing 11, 12, 65, 149, 170, 179
white papers 101
'whole person' perspective 201
Winterbourne View 170
work-life balance 53, 208
workplace well-being 199
work-related stress 207